STOPPING
Cancer
at the
Source

Other books by M. Sara Rosenthal

The Thyroid Sourcebook (4th edition, 2000)
The Gynecological Sourcebook (3rd edition, 1999)
The Pregnancy Sourcebook (3rd edition, 1999)
The Fertility Sourcebook (3rd edition, 1999)
The Breastfeeding Sourcebook (3rd edition, 2000)
The Breast Sourcebook (2nd edition, 1999)
The Gastrointestinal Sourcebook (1997; 1998)
Managing Your Diabetes (1998)
Managing Diabetes for Women (1999)
The Type 2 Diabetic Woman (1999)
The Thyroid Sourcebook for Women (1999)
Women and Sadness (2000)
Women and Depression (2000)
50 Ways To Prevent Colon Cancer (2000)
Women of the '60s Turning 50 (2000)
Women and Passion (2000)
50 Ways To Prevent Heart Disease (2000)
50 Ways To Prevent Depression (2001)
50 Ways To Manage Type 2 Diabetes (2001)
50 Ways To Prevent and Manage Stress (2001)
The Canadian Diabetes Sourcebook (2001)

STOPPING
Cancer
at the
Source

M. Sara Rosenthal

Foreword by Irving Rootman, Ph.D.

Director, University of Toronto Centre for Health Promotion,
a WHO-collaborating centre in health promotion

First published in Canada in 2001 by
Your Health Press™, a division of Sarahealth.com Inc.
in association with Trafford Publishing.

Cover and text design by P. Krulicki, Colborne Communications

National Library of Canada Cataloguing in Publication Data

Rosenthal, M. Sara.
    Stopping cancer at the source

    ISBN 1-55212-746-X

    1. Cancer--Prevention. I. Title.
RC268.R67 2001   616.99'4052   C2001-910672-6

Your Health Press™
A division of Sarahealth.com Inc.
Printed in Canada

IMPORTANT NOTICE

*The purpose of this book is to educate. It is sold with the understanding that the author shall
have neither liability nor responsibility for any injury caused or alleged to be caused directly
or indirectly by the information contained in this book. While every effort has been made to
ensure its accuracy, the book's contents should not be construed as medical advice. Each
person's health needs are unique. To obtain recommendations appropriate to your particular
situation, please consult a qualified health care provider.*

This book was published *on-demand* in cooperation with Trafford Publishing.
On-demand publishing is a unique process and service of making a book available for retail
sale to the public taking advantage of on-demand manufacturing and Internet marketing.
On-demand publishing includes promotions, retail sales, manufacturing, order fulfilment,
accounting and collecting royalties on behalf of the author.

Suite 6E, 2333 Government St., Victoria, B.C. V8T 4P4, CANADA
Phone   250-383-6864   Toll-free   1-888-232-4444 (Canada & US)
Fax   250-383-6804   E-mail   sales@trafford.com
Web site   www.trafford.com   TRAFFORD PUBLISHING IS A DIVISION OF TRAFFORD HOLDINGS LTD.
Trafford Catalogue #01-0146   www.trafford.com/robots/01-0146.html

10   9   8   7   6   5   4   3

In memory of Oscar Welsher
1963–1999

Contents

Preface

IF YOU'RE AMERICAN - READ ME!

Greetings to all my American readers. The information in this book is based on the only comprehensive government report ever produced on how to stop cancer at the source (known as primary prevention of cancer) within North America. It is the only report based on existing science, and written by a cross-section of North American cancer experts who reached consensus over its content. This report did not originate in the United States, but in Canada, with the Ontario government, which declined to use the recommendations in the report. Ontario is where you'll be if you proceed north of Buffalo, New York. It straddles Lake Ontario, one of the Great Lakes. It is a huge, industrial Canadian province that is home to roughly 12 million people. The city of Toronto, which is the capital city of Ontario, boasts a population of more than four million people. So when you think about Ontario, imagine a place very much affected by urban sprawl, with enough cars, industry, pollution, different cultures and communities to look like any large U.S. state. I'm telling you all of this because the information in this book is designed for Anyplace, North America. It is not information about Canada, but about North America. This book also has crucial information from the Eighth Biennial Report on Great Lakes Water Quality, published by the International Joint Commission, 1996, a U.S.-Canada joint document, and the Executive Report of the Environmental Defense Fund, 1997, a U.S. document. The United States and Canada share the same resources, air, and soil. Canada is the United States' largest trading partner. We're in this together. So please join me in reading about what we can do to stop cancer at the source—in both our nations.

Foreword

In late 1994, I was approached by the office of the Ontario Minister of Health to see if the Centre for Health Promotion would be willing to organize a task force that would offer scientifically based advice to the government on the primary prevention of cancer. I accepted this challenge and the first thing I did to fulfill it was to ask Dr. Tony Miller, an internationally acknowledged cancer epidemiologist, to chair the group. Fortunately, he accepted and together we carefully selected the other members of the Task Force on the Primary Prevention of Cancer to represent a broad range of scientific, as well as public, perspectives, including those of cancer survivors. We were successful in appointing an outstanding group of individuals to the Task Force, all of whom approached the work with knowledge, commitment and energy. This resulted in the production of a non-partisan report to the government in March 1995 (perhaps a record time for a government-commissioned task force!).

Unfortunately, the government changed shortly thereafter before action could be taken to implement the recommendations. And as is often the case with changes in government, the report got lost in the shuffle. Thus, when I was approached by community activists about a year later and asked what actions had been taken on the recommendations by the government, we found that very little, if any, changes had occurred. Moreover, it appeared as if the government was not interested in giving the report a high profile, or in moving quickly to implement the recommendations.

This made it quite clear that if anything was going to happen, it would have to come from other sources. Fortunately, there were others who were willing to move the cancer prevention agenda forward. They included a member of the Task Force who was the Medical Officer of Health in London, Ontario, who helped to establish a Cancer Prevention Coalition in that city. It has become a model followed by other communities in Ontario, including Windsor, Kingston and Toronto. They also included activists in Hamilton, Ontario, who organized a conference on cancer prevention that led to the establishment of an Ontario-wide organization, called StopCancer.Ont, committed to primary prevention. In these efforts as well as others, the Task Force Report was used as the guiding framework.

This book is another example of the use of the Report to advance cancer prevention. The idea for such a book emerged out of an Interest Group on the Primary Prevention of Cancer sponsored by the Centre for Health Promotion that also was established to pursue the implementation of the recommendations of the Task Force. It was suggested by that group that it would be extremely helpful if someone was willing to write a book for the general public that made the findings of the Task Force more generally available. Fortunately, Sara Rosenthal, a successful and talented author of numerous books on health topics for the public and a member of the group, was willing to act on this suggestion and was able to publish the book under her own imprint, Your Health Press™.

The net result is the book that you hold in your hands: *Stopping Cancer at the Source*.

You have made an excellent choice in picking up this book and I hope that you will read it from cover to cover as I have done. In addition to strongly making the case for cancer prevention, it offers practical ideas that people like yourself can put into action. This is extremely important given that it is clear that we cannot rely entirely on our governments to prevent cancer. Effective prevention in fact requires action by governments, businesses, universities, voluntary organizations and individuals. This books shows you how to do your part and encourage others to do theirs.
Irving Rootman, Ph.D.,
Director, Centre for Health Promotion

Acknowledgements

First and foremost, this book would not have come to fruition without the unwavering support of Dr. Irving Rootman, Director, University of Toronto Centre for Health Promotion; Ruth Grier, Ontario Minister of the Environment and then Ontario Minister of Health (1990–1995); Dr. Dorothy Goldin-Rosenberg, Women's Network on Health and the Environment, and co-producer, *Exposure: Environmental Links to Breast Cancer*; Maureen Harmer, RN, BScN, MS, Program Manager, Hamilton-Wentworth Regional Public Health Department; Margaret Black, RN, Ph.D., Associate Professor, School of Nursing, McMaster University; as well as all the members of the Cancer Prevention Interest Group at the University of Toronto Centre for Health Promotion, including, especially, Roger Dixon, Industrial Hygienist.

I also wish to thank the original members of the Ontario Task Force on the Primary Prevention of Cancer, whose published recommendations in March 1995 form the framework for this book (listed alphabetically, with their titles at the time of their participation in the report): Dr. Norman Boyd, Division of Epidemiology, Ontario Cancer Institute, and Division of Preventive Oncology, Ontario Cancer Treatment and Research Foundation; the late Dr. Kenneth Carroll, Centre for Human Nutrition, Division of Biochemistry, University of Western Ontario; Dr. William K. Evans, Ontario Cancer Treatment and Research Foundation, Ottawa; Dr. Walter Ewing, Simcoe County District Health Unit, Barrie; Dr. Roberta Ferrence, Ontario Tobacco Research Unit, Addiction Research Foundation, Toronto; Dr. Norman Giesbrecht, Social and Evaluation Research, Addiction Research Foundation, Toronto; Dr. James Gowing, Cambridge Memorial Hospital, Cambridge; Dr. Trevor Hancock, Kleinberg; Dr. Donald Iverson, Behavioural Research and Program Evaluation, National Cancer Institute of Canada,

Toronto; Jeanne Jabanoski, Environmental Protection Office, City of Toronto, Department of Public Health; M. David Kassirer, Toronto; Marilyn Mackenzie, Canadian Cancer Society, Toronto; Dr. Anthony Miller, Chair, Department of Preventive Medicine and Biostatistics, University of Toronto; Dr. David Muir, Occupational Health Program, McMaster University; Dr. Grahame Owen, Oakville; Dr. Graham Pollet, Middlesex–London Health Unit, London; Dr. Irving Rootman, Director, University of Toronto Centre for Health Promotion; Dr. Beth Savan, Environmental Health Program, Innis College, University of Toronto; Dr. Richard Schabas, Public Health Branch, Ontario Ministry of Health; Jack Shapiro, Ontario Cancer Treatment and Research Foundation, Toronto; Marion Stevens, Toronto. *Ex officio Members of the Task Force:* Charles Clayton, Health Promotion Branch, Ministry of Health; Dr. Les Levin, Policy, Programs and Research Branch, Ontario Ministry of Health, Toronto; Dr. Sandy Nuttall, Policy Programs and Research Branch, Ontario Ministry of Health, Toronto; Adam Socha, Ontario Ministry of Environment and Energy, Toronto. *Resource Staff:* Brian Hyndman, Addiction Research Foundation, Toronto, Phil Regli, Policy and Programs Division, Ministry of Agriculture, Food and Rural Affairs, Toronto.

A number of medical advisers who helped me on previous works also helped me to shape much of the content for this book. And so I wish to thank the following people: Gillian Arsenault, M.D., C.C.F.P., I.B.L.C., F.R.C.P.; Pamela Craig, M.D., F.A.C.S., Ph.D.; Masood Kahthamee, M.D., F.A.C.O.G.; Gary May, M.D., F.R.C.P.; James McSherry, M.D., Ch.B., F.C.F.P., F.C.F.P., F.R.C.G.P., F.A.A.F.P., F.A.B.M.P.; Suzanne Pratt, M.D., F.A.C.O.G.; Wm Warren Rudd, M.D., Colon and Rectal Surgeon and Founder and Director of The Rudd Clinic for Diseases of the Colon and Rectum, Toronto; and Robert Volpe, M.D., F.R.C.P., F.A.C.P.

William Harvey, Ph.D., L.L.B., University of Toronto Joint Centre for Bioethics, whose devotion to bioethics has inspired me, continues to support my work and makes it possible for me to have the courage to question and challenge issues in health care and medical ethics. Larissa Kostoff, Editorial Director, Your Health Press™, worked very hard to make this book come into being, as did Laura Tulchinsky, Director, Marketing and Promotion, Your Health Press™. Thanks to Liba Berry for her meticulous copyedit. And finally, Susan Girvan, my consulting editor, made many wonderful and thoughtful suggestions to help make this book informative and incisive.

Introduction

WHO CARES ABOUT STOPPING CANCER AT THE SOURCE?

My friend Tanya cares. Tanya is my best friend. She was widowed at the age of 36 and left with two small children to raise. Her husband Oscar, also 36, was diagnosed with advanced esophageal cancer in May 1999, and was dead by Halloween of that year. The oncologist who diagnosed him told him, "There's nothing we can do; look into alternatives." Abandoned by the traditional medical community, Tanya, Oscar and their families scrambled in all directions, trying detoxifying diets, meditation, supplements and vitamins by the dozen, and newfangled, expensive treatments in a race against the clock. The more they read and educated themselves about Oscar's cancer, the angrier they became.

Why does a strong, healthy, 36-year-old man get cancer? What did this? Tanya then began fearing for her children's health: were they safe from cancer? How could she protect them from the same disease? Or herself, for that matter? The truth is, most people don't really care about cancer prevention until someone they love suffers or dies from it. In Oscar's case, there are no known prevention tactics for esophageal cancer, which accounts for only 2 percent of all cancers and is more common in men over age 60 who smoke and drink. But Oscar does not fit into those criteria. Was he possibly exposed to a carcinogenic toxin, a cancer-causing chemical that was airborne or in the water that he drank? An oncologist may say he was genetically predisposed, which means he was wired for certain cancers at birth, and something tripped the switch. Indeed, we are all wired for hundreds of potential diseases and cancers, and some people may be more wired than others. In order to stop cancer at the source, we need to look at what's turning on those switches.

Stopping Cancer at the Source

I was diagnosed with thyroid cancer at the age of 20, a cancer that, prior to the 1980s, was rare in young people. Because of radiaoactive fallout from nuclear testing, many young adults, teens and children are developing thyroid cancer. In fact, thyroid cancer is epidemic in Eastern Europe, and often incurable in those regions due to a more aggressive strain of that particular cancer. In my case, there wasn't anything I could have done to prevent my cancer, since I was exposed to an airborne carcinogen. Unless I could have personally stopped nuclear testing and fallout, I could not have prevented my cancer.

What should infuriate you are the deaths from cancers that could have been stopped at the source. What about people who die from lung cancer, when most lung cancer would never occur were it not for the aggressive marketing of tobacco products? Or colon cancer, when colon cancer is preventable through diet and lifestyle changes? Or melanoma, when more information about sun safety could have prevented death?

Much of the information in this book is based on the *Report of the Ontario Task Force on the Primary Prevention of Cancer*. Ontario, Canada's most populous and industrial province, saw in the late 1980s that it was in trouble when it came to cancer—it has too much of it for its health care system to handle. Designed to address the burgeoning issue of a cancer epidemic in the face of an ageing population and dramatic cuts to Canada's health care system, the task force was appointed February 1994 by Ruth Grier, then the Ontario Minister of Health. It was chaired by Dr. Anthony Miller, chair of the Department of Preventive Medicine and Biostatistics at the University of Toronto. A key representative of the Ministry of Health was Dr. Les Levin, a supporter of primary cancer prevention and Service Adviser on Cancer Policy for the ministry. The Task Force Report was facilitated by the director of the University of Toronto's Centre for Health Promotion, Dr. Irving Rootman. An interdisciplinary team of environmental scientists, oncologists and activists from across Ontario put thousands of hours into the report.

The Ontario government was voted out of power shortly after the report's release; the new government wanted to grow business, and failed to act on its recommendations. What you're about to read is what the Ontario government was told in 1995 that it should do, based on a review of existing science and a report written by consensus. This book gives you the real tools you need to act to prevent cancer. As I've stressed in this book's preface, you don't have to live in Ontario, Canada to benefit from the information and suggestions contained here; they are designed for residents of

Anyplace, North America. It is the definitive book on stopping cancer for Joe and Jane Q. Public.

I have made the Task Force Report accessible by translating the technical information it contains into plain language. I have also added to the original report information from the *Eighth Biennial Report on Great Lakes Water Quality,* published by the International Joint Commission, 1996, and the *Executive Report of the Environmental Defense Fund,* 1997. I also used material from the Government of Canada's State of Knowledge Report on Environmental Contaminants and Human Health in the Great Lakes Basin (1997). Included here as well are the recommendations and suggestions made in collaboration with experts in cancer prevention, which have been added since the original report was released. Finally, I have provided you with prevention information that was not in the original report, based on my own body of research as a medical journalist and my work in bioethics.

This is a book about stopping cancer at the source, also known as the primary prevention of cancer. The term "primary prevention" refers to preventing a disease at its origins. There's a world of difference between the terms "prevention" and "detection." There is also a vast difference between primary prevention and secondary prevention. When the medical community discusses "cancer prevention," it usually means cancer detection through screening or other diagnostic tests, or by self-exam; meanwhile, prescribing drugs to prevent a certain cancer is a form of secondary prevention. But primary prevention means changing the behavior that causes the disease, or eliminating the carcinogen responsible for the disease. For example, if smoking is responsible for most lung cancers, not smoking can stop lung cancer at the source. On the food and drink front, we know that a host of carcinogens are fat-soluble, so by making our bodies leaner through diet and exercise, we can possibly stop other kinds of cancers at the source.

The information contained in this book is supported by accepted scientific evidence and studies.* Where the evidence is incomplete or unknown, this book tells you so. A complete list of the original sources used to compile the Task Force Report is included in the bibliography.

It is hoped that the ideas contained in these pages will inspire public protest and help initiate the policy changes that scientists and public health advocates have been demanding since the late twentieth century. If you have been diagnosed with cancer and are looking for treatment information, this is not the book for you; if someone you love has died or suffered from cancer, this is the book I hope you read.

If one child is spared a cancer diagnosis in adulthood as a result of information in this book, all of the efforts of all the individuals who contributed to the Task Force Report on which this book is based will have been worth it. As the Talmudic saying goes: "S/he who saves a life eventually saves the world."

* Note: The evidence is accurate as of statistics available during this writing. New information will continually be made available, which will back up much of what is reported in this book, or answer questions we don't know the answers to right now. Indeed, the evidence and studies in this area have just begun, and will continue long into this century. The information contained in this book is the best start we have right now, and is designed to inspire you to do further investigation into cancer prevention. Stay in touch with me through my website at *www.sarahealth.com*. Together, we will add to this book in future updates.

1
WHAT IS CANCER?

Cancer is the general term for the abnormal growth of cells. When the abnormal cell reproduces, it has the ability to invade or metastasize to other parts of the body. The actual word "cancer" is Latin for crab. It was, in fact, the crab-like appearance of advanced breast tumors that inspired the Roman physician Galen to name cancer. In Greek, "karkinos" originally meant "crab," too, which is how Hippocrates first identified and classified this illness 2500 years ago.

Cancer was an extremely rare disease in the ancient world, and is not mentioned at all in the Bible or the *Yellow Emperor's Classic of Internal Medicine,* the ancient medicine book of China. It began to be seen more extensively around the time of the Industrial Revolution.

Actually, the cancer cell itself is not dangerous (unlike bacteria or viruses), but its impact on the rest of the organs is. As it spreads into various parts of the body, it interferes with the jobs of regular cells, confuses other organs, and can wreak havoc. It's basically a terrorist cell, hijacking organs and other cells. Cancer cells use the lymph system to get into the bloodstream and then travel throughout the body. These cells love organs that have multiple blood vessels and nutrients, such as bones, lungs and brains—common areas where cancer spreads.

Cancer cells are divided into two groups: carcinoma and sarcoma. A carcinoma refers to cancerous cells made of epithelial cells—cells that line various tissues. You'll find carcinomas in organs that tend to secrete something (milk, mucus, digestive juices, and so on). Common sites for carcinomas are breasts, lungs and colons. Carcinomas account for 80–90 percent of all human cancers, and are generally slow-growing. There is always a prefix attached to the word "carcinoma" that will tell us where the carcinoma is growing, and the kinds of cells that are involved. An adenocarcinoma, for example, is a carcinoma made of glandular cells. When you just see the word "oma" by itself, it means benign. An adenoma refers to a clump of benign glandular cells; a fibroma refers to a clump of benign fibrous cells, and so on. When the cells are malignant, the word carcinoma is attached to the end, as in adenocarcinoma. It gets even more specific. You'll need to know where the adenocarcinoma itself originated. Think of it like this: carcinoma used by itself is as descriptive as saying "sweater." Adenocarcinoma is like saying "wool sweater." More specific descriptions can be "lambswool sweater" or "angora sweater." And there can be other prefixes that are synonymous with saying "blue angora sweater." There are literally hundreds of carcinomas, all described by a different combination of prefixes identifying the parts of the bodies that are involved, the shape of the carcinomas, etc.

Sarcomas are cancerous cells made up of supporting connective tissue. Sarcomas are rare and account for only 2 percent of all human cancers but tend to be more aggressive than carcinomas. Again, the prefixes before the word tell you where the sarcoma is located, what it's made of, what shape it is, etc., while sometimes sarcomas are named after the doctors who discovered them. Just like above, the word "oma" in Sarcomaspeak means benign. The difference between a carcinoma and a sarcoma is equal to the difference between a sweater and a boot; both are different things, but related. Nonetheless, both have different physical properties, are made of different materials, available in different colors, and so on. (You can also have a carcinosarcoma—a carcinoma and sarcoma all in one.)

Since cancer cells are living cells, it's in their nature to continue to live. So the first thing cancer cells do is grow. They'll simply begin growing where they first originated, be it the lung or colon. The second thing cancer cells do is change. They mutate from the other cells that surround them. After they get to a certain age they want to move out and leave their original nest. So they spread out into surrounding fat and tissue.

A very crucial motive of the cancer cell is to eat. So the cancer cell sends out protein messengers (called tumor angiogenesis factors) that create new blood vessels to feed it. If a cancer cell can manage these four basic functions, it will live, and we'll experience the result of this in the form of a tumor. If any of these functions is stopped, the cancer will die. As you've guessed by now, treatments will therefore attempt to interfere with these four functions. These treatments aim to: stop the cells from growing; stop the cells from changing or mutating; stop the cells from spreading; or stop the cells from eating.

If the cancer continues to live, it will simply continue these same basic behaviors: it will grow bigger; change and mutate even more to trick the immune system; and spread out even more by bursting into surrounding structures and into the blood vessels. Finally, if the cells reach adulthood, they'll want to settle down and find a good home, preferably an organ with a lining in its blood vessels, like liver, lungs and bone. So the cells attach to these blood vessels, and pass through them into such an organ. And they will continue to make themselves comfortable so they can reproduce more and more. This means setting themselves up with a new blood supply to make the organ more conducive to their growth. And so it goes, until the cancer occupies every space in the body. The most important thing to remember is that none of this happens immediately; it can take years for these cancer cells to really spread.

In Situ vs. Invasive

Regardless of whether the cancer is a carcinoma or sarcoma of some kind, the most important words are these: *in situ* and *invasive. In situ* means "in one place." A carcinoma *in situ* means that the carcinoma is confined to a specific area and has not spread. This is good news and means that the cancer is, by definition, non-invasive and is in an early stage. Invasive carcinoma means that the cancer has spread to local tissue, surrounding tissue, lymph nodes or other organs. This is not good news and means that the cancer is in a later stage. However, even though a cancer may be invasive and in a later stage, it can still mean that it is quite treatable.

Differentiated vs. Undifferentiated

Cancer cells are classified into two behavioral categories: differentiated and undifferentiated. These terms refer to the sophistication of the cancer cells. Differentiated cancer cells resemble the cells of their origin. A differentiated cancer cell that originates in the colon, for example, would look and act like a normal colon cell. In fact, these cancer cells might actually assist the other cells with routine functions. Because these cells spend some of their time assisting the body, they spend less time reproducing, and therefore take a lot longer to metastasize or spread to other parts of the body. But both differentiated and undifferentiated cells are equally treatable; key factors are tumor size and lymph node status. Often, you won't find a purely differentiated cell. It may look just moderately abnormal. Because of this, there are subclassifications: moderately differentiated, well differentiated or poorly differentiated. These classifications are known as the cells' *grading*. A high grade means that the cell is immature, poorly differentiated and therefore faster growing; a low grade cancer cell is mature, well-differentiated, slow growing and less aggressive. However, this is a terribly basic explanation of cell grading, something which is based on far more complex criteria.

Undifferentiated cancer is made up of very primitive cells that look wild and untamed, bearing little or no resemblance to the cells of origin. They don't assist the body at all, and are therefore able to spend all of their time reproducing. This is more dangerous because the cells may then spread faster. There are cases, though, when undifferentiated cancer is not very aggressive, despite the fact that it involves more primitive cells. In these cases, the cancer looks wilder than it behaves. This is often the case in breast cancers.

There are also mixes of these different cells, which affect the aggressiveness of the disease. For example, there can be mostly differentiated cells mixed in with a few undifferentiated cells, or vice versa. Whatever is most abundant will affect the behavior of the cancer; mostly differentiated cells will slow down whatever undifferentiated cells exist, while mostly undifferentiated cells will speed up whatever differentiated cells exist.

How Cancer Starts

One theory is that every individual has certain oncogenes that remain dormant in the body until an external agent turns them on—like a switch. Once turned on, the oncogene is responsible for transforming normal cells into abnormal cells. But what trips one person's cancer switch, however, may not trip someone else's cancer switch, which may be why some people get cancer, while others do not. So in this sense, while it's believed that cancers are genetic, it's also believed that external or environmental factors are responsible for triggering them.

Here's one way to think about it: we may all have some sort of weapon inside of us. Some of us have .38 caliber pistols; some of us have Uzis; some of us have cannons, and so on. But the cells that pull the trigger only do so when repeatedly provoked by outside forces like tobacco, X-rays, excess estrogen, sunlight, radioactive fallout or industrial agents. So while one cigarette may irritate lung cells, 20 years of smoking may provide multiple hits to these cells, hits that finally provoke them to pull the trigger.

What is Your Cancer Risk?

How to assess your cancer risk is probably the foremost question on your mind now. This chapter is designed to help you answer that question, so you can put a lot of the "What's Personal" information into action.

What Cancers Can You Stop at the Source?

The recipe for stopping cancer at the source on the personal front is remembering this "holy trinity":

1. Health enhancement. This entails eating well and staying physically active, as well as practicing proper hygiene and safe sex. It also means staying mentally and spiritually fit, which reduces stress and boosts the immune system. Choose health. As consumer demand goes up, more healthy products will become available at reasonable prices. This also includes healthy products for the earth and environment.

2. Risk avoidance. This means avoiding bad things, or known carcinogens, such as tobacco, excessive alcohol or even low-nutrient foods, such as junk foods with empty calories and no nutrients. It also means finding out about local environmental conditions in your workplace or community and avoiding clear hazards where you can.

3. Risk reduction. This means lowering your exposure to something you can't help being exposed to, such as occupational toxins; or wearing protective masks or clothing; or choosing organic produce over pesticide-laden produce; or choosing clean water over contaminated water. Lobbying for better products, services, policies and by-laws are all part of risk reduction.

As noted, we're all born with a big "basement light switch" that is wired for potential diseases, including certain cancers. At birth, all of these switches are off. As we age and indulge in certain diets, habits or activities or are exposed to certain toxins through work or lifestyle choices, these switches can be turned on. Nobody knows which switches are being turned on at certain points. All we can do is try to eliminate the triggers that can change our switches from off to on. Any cancer that is linked to the following can be stopped at the source through lifestyle modification that involves a combination of health enhancement, risk avoidance or risk reduction tactics:

- Smoking, substance or alcohol abuse (chapters 2 and 3)
- Poor, high-fat, low-nutrient diets (chapter 3)
- Sedentary or inactive lifestyle (chapter 4)
- Exposure to sun damage (chapter 5)

A Summary of Risk Factors

In order to practice health enhancement, risk avoidance or risk reduction, you need to understand what is really meant by the phrase "risk factors." What does it mean when you're told you're "at risk" for a particular cancer—or any other disease? A few things, depending on the adjective that precedes the word "risk."

When trying to understand risk factors, having a degree in actuarial science really helps. That's because there is a world of difference between absolute, cumulative, relative and attributable risk. Absolute risk means that the cancer rate is counted in numbers of cases occurring within a group of people. When you hear, for example, that in the town of Anywhere, "50 out of 100,000 people died last year of a particular cancer," this is absolute risk. The official definition of absolute risk is "the observed or calculated probability of an event in a population under study." So this can be a hypothetical or real population; it's just not relative to any other population.

Cumulative risk just means "added up." It's a risk per unit of time added up over X units of time, such as a lifetime or a given time frame that a study ran, such as 2 years or 10 years. It can be an estimate or the experiences of a real group of people—but it will be an average of the experiences of that group. So when you see "cumulative risk factors," it is a "guess" of risk based on a number of factors that may include mortalities from a particular cancer in a given area or age group and mortalities of people who share your same medical history. So cumulative risk is not based on you, personally, but on estimates. It's like betting in a horse race. You look at the ages of the horses, the histories, the breeding, the jockeys and where the race is being run, and you come up with odds. When you read, for example, that "one in eight people over a lifetime" will get a particular cancer, this is a cumulative risk—an average, not an absolute. The problem with a statement like that is that it tends to underestimate risk in some, while overestimating risk in others.

Then there's relative risk, which is based on comparing two populations. For example, when people who eat large amounts of fat are at greater risk for certain cancers than people who have low-fat diets, this refers to relative risk. It directly compares a population that has one type of risk factor with a population that has a different risk factor. It basically compares risk in situation A with risk in situation B (which is usually a standard or constant, such as "no risk factor").

But this doesn't mean that people who eat large amounts of fat cannot alter their diets, or people who smoke cannot quit smoking. When you speak of risk that can be reduced, prevented or altered through behavior (like quitting smoking or dieting), you're now talking about modifiable risk because it is under voluntary control. This is different from a "risk marker," such as family history, which cannot be modified. It is also different from attributable risk, which refers to a component of one's risk attributable to either a modifiable risk factor, such as diet, or a risk marker, such as family history.

Not all cancers can be linked to an absolute cause either. For example, breast cancer is not like lung cancer. With lung cancer, we know that at least 70 percent of those who develop it smoke. Therefore, you can absolutely say that smoking causes lung cancer, a cancer that kills more people each year than any other cancer. You can't name one main cause of breast cancer, however. All you can do is count up the people who are diagnosed with the disease, examine the kinds of lifestyles or family histories they have that may be different from those of people without breast cancer, and analyze the effects of each type of difference.

What most of us have been bombarded with since the 1970s are the reports of known risk factors for certain cancers. It's important to understand that many of the "known" risks are conflicting and often controversial. While one study suggests that this or that increases your risk of some cancer, another study may suggest the contrary.

Statistics are very tricky. For example, if odds are less than 1 in 20 of something being found by chance, it's said to be "statistically significant." For example, a certain characteristic, such as eye colour, makes absolutely no difference to anybody's chance of getting a particular cancer. Yet for every 20 studies or comparisons done on this characteristic, one of those studies might show a "significant" departure from the conclusion of "no difference" between cases of people with a particular cancer and the control group (people without that particular cancer). When you see the phrase "statistically significant" in the newspaper, remember that it may mean "we found this purely by chance," even though the media may be going wild. The bottom line is that you have to be careful not to jump to conclusions when you hear breaking news about a new risk. That said, it's important to understand that no one, single risk factor, such as age or diet, can be interpreted as an absolute cause of most cancers. As mentioned earlier, there are many lifestyle changes you can make to significantly lower your risks. In addition, understanding the environmental impact on many cancers will help you put these risks in perspective.

Another final distinction is the difference between association and causation. When you see a statement like "Men with prostate cancer were found to eat more fat than men without prostate cancer," this means association. It does not mean that dietary fat causes prostate cancer. When you see the sentence "Smoking causes lung cancer," this is an example of causation.

The following is an alphabetical list of common, known risk factors for various cancers. The risk factors you can change (avoid or reduce) have an asterisk by the heading.

Age
The risk of many cancers is largely age-related because so much cancer is dependent on our behaviors (diet, activity, etc.). The tendency is for most cancers to strike over age 45. When young adults or children develop cancer, it is usually due to exposure to a carcinogen or toxin; in rare cases, there are inherited cancers that strike people at young ages.

*Bad Habits**
Any lifestyle indulgence that has proven risk factors is, for the purpose of this book, considered a bad habit. If you smoke, drink an excessive amount of alcohol or abuse illegal drugs, your risk of getting some diseases is higher than it is for people who don't do these things.

Geographics
Who gets cancer largely depends on where people live. Many cancers are "regional." For example, industrialized countries have much higher rates of certain cancers than underdeveloped countries. Region dramatically affects the rates of many cancers, and we just don't know why. For instance, the breast cancer rate in Geneva is double that of Spain—even though the two countries are not that far apart geographically. In San Francisco, the rate of breast cancer is double that of Newfoundland, proving that breast cancer in North America can vary from coast to coast.

People emigrating from regions with low rates of certain cancers increase their own risk when they enter a country with higher incidences of those cancers, which suggests that many cancers are largely caused by environmental factors, such as lifestyle, culture, diet, water and air quality.

*Diet**

Diet, as discussed in chapter 3, plays an enormous role in cancer risk.

Environmental Factors
Environmental factors are extremely important when assessing your risk of cancer, as discussed in chapters 7 through 9.

Estrogen
High levels of estrogen seem to be markers for increased risk of reproductive cancers, such as breast and endometrial. Sources of extra estrogen include:

- Exposure to DES (diethylstilbestrol), a drug administered to pregnant women from the 1940s to the 1970s to supposedly stop miscarriage. DES daughters are at risk for a variety of reproductive cancers, mainly vaginal and cervical.
- Birth control pills
- Fertility drugs
- Hormone replacement therapy (HRT)
- Body fat (This is not an external source of estrogen, but may contribute to your fat cells' production of estrogen if the fat you eat makes you fat!)
- Environmental estrogens (see chapter 8)
- Hormone-fed produce

Exercise Habits*
Sedentary living breeds ill health and is associated with higher rates of many cancers, as discussed in chapter 4.

Family History
As discussed in chapter 6, we are all vulnerable to some diseases more than others.

Education, Income and Cancer Risk

Not all of us have access to the kind of information or the kind of services we need to stay healthy. Some of this inequality is based on income; some is based on education and literacy. Studies that review what we call "socio-economic determinants" always find the same thing. The poorer the population, the more disease. Seniors living on fixed incomes, disadvantaged minority or aboriginal populations often do not have access to the right information to stay healthy.

Stopping Cancer at the Source

It's been demonstrated time and time again that low-income individuals do not enjoy the same quality of health as their more fortunate neighbors. For example, a study linking life expectancy to neighborhood income found that men living in the wealthiest districts lived an average of 5.7 years longer than men from the poorest neighborhoods, while the average lifespan for women from the richest neighborhoods was almost 2 years longer than their low-income counterparts. All of the factors discussed in Part 1 of this book, such as good diet with access to nutritious foods, as well as physical activity, are also rich versus poor issues. The rich can afford better food than the poor; the rich have more leisure time than the poor.

In chapter 7 you'll read about occupational hazards. Well, there again you'll see that occupational cancers are more prevalent among blue-collar workers and non-unionized laborers.

We also know that contaminated areas in North America are often inhabited by those with low incomes. Quite simply, many can't afford to leave areas that have become contaminated, while poorer communities tend to be the ones that are home to contaminated waste, landfills and so on.

Poor nutrition, occupational hazards, lack of access to good screening tests or health care counseling, stress associated with being poor (this is not insignificant, by the way), "self medicating" through addictions such as smoking and alcohol consumption all play a role in cancer incidence. This may be one reason cancer hits harder in low-income neighborhoods. Evidence shows that specific cancers reveal considerable differences in the incidence and mortality rates of the rich and the poor.

Low socio-economic status is associated with higher incidence of, and mortality from, the following:

- Stomach cancer;
- Lung cancer in men;
- Cervical cancer; and
- Cancers of the mouth, pharynx, larynx and esophagus.

Higher-income groups don't get away scot-free, because there are certain cancers that are linked to "luxury" or "opportunity." These cancers are influenced by higher-fat diets, less physical activity (more cars), and more vacations in the sun.

High socio-economic status is associated with a higher incidence of, and mortality from, the following:

- Skin cancer;

- Breast cancer;
- Prostate cancer; and
- Colon cancer in men.

As you look at this list, it's easy to see how lifestyle habits affect certain groups. Looking at the "wealthy" cancers: colon, breast and prostate cancers are associated with too much fat (often because of privileged diets), too much driving and not enough physical activity; skin cancer is associated with vacation and leisure time in the sun. So, when it comes to tracking the incidence of disease, it's important to remember that socio-economic differences often bring with them corresponding differences in health-related behaviors, such as smoking, alcohol consumption and eating habits. Reducing the much higher rates of smoking among economically disadvantaged groups is perhaps our biggest task in bringing about a reduction in socio-economic inequities in health status. All lifestyle behaviors have to be looked at in the context of the social, economic, environmental and political factors that motivate them, and that act, in many cases, as barriers to the maintenance of good health.

As stated throughout this book, cancer is caused by many different things, which probably converge. But there are clearly certain carcinogens that cause certain cancers, such as tobacco, which causes lung cancer. We also know that enhancing our health through nutritious food and regular exercise is definitely associated with lower rates of many cancers. Lean bodies provide less fat in which fat-soluble carcinogens can live, while high-fiber diets and exercise are essential for colon health

PART I

WHAT'S PERSONAL

Stopping Cancer at the Source

The good news is that altering your personal lifestyle habits can stop cancer at the source. The top two killer cancers for both sexes are lung and colon cancer. How can lifestyle changes alter this grim fact? By not smoking, and by reducing your exposure to second-hand smoke, you can stop lung cancer at the source (chapter 2). By adopting a high-fiber diet that is low in fat, and by incorporating activity into your daily routine, you can help to stop colon and other cancers at the source (chapters 3 and 4). Staying lean will also help reduce your exposure to fat-soluble toxins—toxic substances that set up house within your fat cells. Staying lean will also help reduce your risk of contracting estrogen-dependent cancers, such as breast, colon, ovarian and endometrial cancers, because it is fat that produces estrogen. Moreover, practicing sun safety can also help to stop skin cancers at the source (chapter 5).

Also within your personal control are cancers known to be caused by sexually transmitted diseases (STDs). These include cervical cancer (which can be caught early through routine Pap tests), female genital cancers (vaginal and vulvar), and cancer of the penis in men. (Prostate and testicular cancers are not considered "genital" cancers.) By simply practicing safe sex (this information is available in my books *The Gynecological Sourcebook*, 3rd edition and *The Fertility Sourcebook*), you can stop these cancers at the source, too. Since safe sex information is widely available, I've decided not to include a chapter on it to make space for information you won't find anywhere else.

A frank discussion with your health care provider about your cancer risk and the various medications you may be taking—especially estrogen-containing medications—is another way of bringing cancer control into your life. Be sure to ask about all known side effects of prescription medications you're taking, and whether those substances conflict with the over-the-counter drugs or herbal products you're taking.

Finally, any female reader concerned specifically about her breast cancer risk, or interested in learning about prevention therapies for breast cancer, should also consult my book *The Breast Sourcebook*, 2nd edition.

2
TOBACCO WARS

I am a diehard non-smoker and am completely frustrated by having smoke continuously blown in my face by passersby on the street or by restaurant patrons still allowed to smoke in public places. Without question, all non-smokers' rights are being violated when they are forced to inhale second-hand smoke. Our children's rights to a healthy environment are being violated by the continued advertising and sale of tobacco; it is our teens who begin smoking, and grow into tobacco and nicotine-addicted adults, who are at high risk of premature death, directly caused by tobacco. And it is our babies and children who suffer the effects of second-hand smoke through respiratory disorders. Moreover, the number of people who die in fires each year caused by burning cigarettes is not insignificant.

It's not news that smoking causes cancer. Countless national and international groups have reviewed the effects of tobacco smoke on health, and the evidence has been in for a long time: smoking tobacco causes cancer in smokers, and exposure to second-hand tobacco smoke causes cancer in non-smokers.

Although the number of smokers in North America has declined substantially over the past 25 years, we still have a long way to go. Studies on tobacco continue to point to the prevalence of smoking among preteens. In fact, more preteens are smoking today than they did in the 1970s. Over 15 percent of youth aged 12–19 years are smokers. Tobacco smoke is the most easily removable cancer-causing agent from our environment. Thus, cancer from smoking remains the most preventable form of cancer and premature mortality. While there are government initiatives in place to ban smoking from more public places throughout North America, there is still not enough support from the public. Only 20 states and Washington, D.C. have laws that restrict smoking in private-sector workplaces; 30 states and Washington, D.C. have laws that restrict smoking in restaurants. In Canada, Toronto and Vancouver (the country's two largest cities) tried to pass laws that would prohibit smoking in all bars and restaurants, to date a success only in Vancouver. One in six premature deaths can be attributed to tobacco use. In addition to heart disease and stroke, lung cancer continued to be the leading cause of cancer deaths among North American women in 1999; statistics from that same year in men reveal that lung cancer follows prostate cancer as the leading cause of cancer deaths.

A host of other cancers are caused by smoking, too. Smokers have a higher risk of developing cancers of the lip, mouth, pharynx, esophagus, bladder, kidneys and pancreas. Smoking has also been linked to an increased risk of cervical cancer. And users of smokeless tobacco products, like chewing tobacco and snuff, have a higher risk of developing cancers of the mouth.

Many cancer deaths will occur in former smokers. Quitting smoking does decrease the odds of getting cancer, but former smokers will always be at higher risk than those who have never smoked. The best way to prevent smoking-associated cancer deaths is never to smoke. And for smokers, the earlier you quit, the greater the benefit.

Carcinogens in Tobacco

In 1989, the U.S. Surgeon General released a report listing 43 carcinogenic agents found in tobacco smoke. The IARC (International Agency for Research on Cancer) classified them as follows:

Group 1A—Carcinogenic to Humans

Tobacco Smoke
Tobacco Products, Smokeless
4-Aminobuphenyl
Benzene
Cadmium
Chromium
2-Naphthylamine
Nickel
Polonium
Nickel
Polonium-210 (Radon)
Vinyl Chloride

Group 2A—Probably Carcinogenic to Humans

Acrylonitrile
Benzo[a]anthracene
Benzo[a]pyrene
1,3-Butadine
Dibenz[a,h]anthracene
Formaldehyde
N-Nitrosodiethylamine
N-Nitrosodimethlamine

Group 2B—Possibly Carcinogenic to Humans

Acetaldehyde
Benzo[b]fluoranthene
Benzo[j]fluoranthene
Benzo[k]fluoranthene
Dibenz[a,h]acridine
Dibenz[a,j-acridine
7H-Dibenz[c,g]carbazole
Dibenzo[a,l]pyrene
1,1-Dimethylhydrazine
Hydrazine
Indeno-2,3-cd]pyrene
Lead
5-Methylchrysene
4-(Methylnitrosamine)
  -2-(3-pyridyl)-1-butanene (NNK)
2-Nitropropane

N-Nitrosodiethanolamine
N-Nitrosomethylethylamine
N-Nitrosomorpholine
N-Nitrosopyrrolidine
Quinoline
Ortho-Toluidine
Urethane (Ethyl Carbamate)

Group 3—Unclassified as to Carcinogenicity to Humans (Limited Evidence)

Chrysene
Crotonaldehyde
N-Nitrosoanabasine (NAB)
N-Nitrosoanatabine (NAT)

ENVIRONMENTAL TOBACCO SMOKE (ETS)

What should really spark some action concerning tobacco and smoking is that non-smokers are vulnerable to tobacco-related cancers. Second-hand smoke, also known as environmental tobacco smoke (ETS), is recognized as a leading cause of lung cancer in non-smokers and respiratory problems in young children and adults. The 1986 report of the U.S. Surgeon General concluded that involuntary exposure to second-hand smoke could cause tobacco-related diseases, including lung cancer. This landmark document proved that no one is without risk, and changed the focus of a decision not to smoke from a lifestyle issue to an environmental health hazard.

Ten years later, a report from the U.S. Environmental Protection Agency (EPA) confirmed the Surgeon General's conclusions by classifying ETS as a Class A carcinogen, the most incriminating category of cancer-causing agents. The report found that ETS, which is a combination of side-stream and exhaled smoke, causes lung cancer in non-smokers and impairs the health of infants and children. To help make all North American public areas smoke-free, we need to support government initiatives rather than fight them. As a non-smoker, the fact that I have to endure smoking sections in restaurants in the twenty-first century is disturbing, considering how easy it is to remove this environmental toxin from the air.

Pregnancy and Infants

Fetuses and children whose parents smoke are the most vulnerable to ETS.

Stopping Cancer at the Source

Respiratory illnesses are more common in children born to smokers, while smoking during pregnancy can lead to the premature rupture of membranes, premature birth, perinatal death, placental abnormalities and bleeding during pregnancy.

Breastfeeding mothers who smoke will find that their milk supply is affected by nicotine (they may make less milk). As a result, they may be depriving their children of the benefits of breastfeeding, and exposing them to the dangers of formula feeding (such as numerous gastro-intestinal problems). The American Academy of Pediatrics lists any amount of nicotine as contraindicated during breastfeeding. Too much nicotine can cause shock, vomiting, diarrhea, rapid heart rate and restlessness in the baby. Second-hand smoke is, arguably, even more damaging to your baby than nicotine levels in breast milk. There are dozens of studies that conclude: "Yes, babies who breathe in smoke from one or both parents don't feel as well as babies born to non-smokers." Second-hand smoke can also cause pneumonia, bronchitis or even SIDS (Sudden Infant Death Syndrome).

Preventing Exposure to ETS

Local governments across North America are struggling to make public areas smoke-free, but they must have public support—*our* support. There are a number of ways you can help. Consider the following ways to avoid or help ban ETS:

- Find out your local government's position on tobacco smoke and let the rest of the government know you support it.
- Stop patronizing restaurants, bars, cafés or smaller businesses that allow smoking, and write to them to let them know that they are losing your business for that precise reason. If you really love the food, suggest smoking sections in a separately ventilated enclosure.
- Name names in letters to the editor or "have-your-say" camera-booth programs; identify smoke-filled restaurants or other businesses and state your reasons for not patronizing them. Negative press works wonders!
- Make a point of congratulating restaurants, bars, cafés or smaller businesses on creating smoke-free environments, and name names to create positive press for their efforts. (I wrote one donut chain a love letter of sorts when I discovered some of their non-smoking locations.)
- Turn in employers who continue to allow smoking in the workplace by

alerting your public health department. You can also sue your employer for tobacco-related disability and ask for compensation for long-term health effects. These suits work best when a group of people sue for the same reason, known as a class action suit.

- If you're concerned about a child of smoking parents, have a friendly chat with the parent in the vein of "Did you know that…" Many smoking parents may not be aware that second-hand smoke is especially concentrated in homes with carpets, or in the family car. Some tact and finesse is necessary here; parents who smoke do not willfully want to damage their children's health!

Cutting Smoke out of Your House
If you live with a smoker or if you smoke in your home, here are some ways to avoid ETS: stop smoking inside the house (go outdoors); create a separate smoking room with its own ventilation system and air seals to keep the smoke out of the other part of the house; install a more effective ventilation system with a supply of outside air and a special filter called a particulate filter.

WAGING WAR ON TOBACCO

The war on tobacco will be won only with individual and community support. Through education, counseling, school and workplace programs, and some anti-smoking legislation, we can have a large impact and help people avoid the effects of tobacco smoke. The goal of anti-tobacco programs is simple: to deter young people from smoking, to encourage smokers to quit, and to protect the public from health risks associated with environmental tobacco smoke.

Raising Tobacco Taxes

If you'd like to see a reduction in smoking, write to your local or federal government and demand that taxes on tobacco be raised to the max. There is strong evidence to suggest that people smoke less when they are forced to pay more for their habit. A good example of this is in Canada: Between 1979 and 1991, Canadian cigarette prices doubled due to federal and provincial tax increases. The added expense was an obvious deterrent: there was a 60 percent drop in the prevalence of smoking among young people. But after 1994, when prices dropped again, making smoking more affordable for teenagers and low-income adults, smoking among young people increased. In short, lower tobacco prices removed the incentive to quit.

Restricting Access to Tobacco Products

Although a minimum age for the purchase of tobacco has been in place for at least a decade in most provinces and states, efforts to enforce these restrictions are usually weak. By imposing fines on retailers who sell cigarettes to minors, and by initiating education programs to make retailers aware of the penalties, as well as the role they can play in preventing teens from smoking in the first place, fewer retailers will continue to sell tobacco to minors, and their access to cigarettes will be further restricted.

Cigarettes ought not be made available everywhere. But in many regions in North America, they are. Our governments could consider licensing all sales outlets, and making it a stiff licensing fee that goes to health care. Alternatively, tobacco products could be made available only through retail outlets controlled by the state or province. In the same way that there are provincially controlled liquor stores in Canada, there could be state-controlled, or provincially controlled tobacco stores, too. Each state or province could establish a Tobacco Control Board or agency, which could assume responsibility for the control of tobacco products and coordinate efforts to limit their availability. As one of its highest priorities such an agency might also have the right to investigate the practices of the tobacco industry. The job of a regulatory commission or board would be to:

- recommend new public policy and report directly to the Department of Health and Human Services in the U.S. or to Health Canada;
- license or control access to tobacco products;
- regulate promotional activities of the tobacco industry;
- enforce cost-recovery methods of smoking-related health costs;
- work with other organizations to develop information and educational strategies;
- assist health professionals and institutions in counseling smokers about methods of quitting; and
- control the export of tobacco products.

Banning Tobacco Advertising and Sponsorship

Tobacco companies should not be allowed to sponsor sports or cultural

Designation of Tobacco as a Hazardous Product

You may have seen some of these product-label warnings: Smoking Causes Lung Cancer; Smoking During Pregnancy Can Harm Your Baby; Smoking May Cause Heart Disease. Ideally, tobacco ought to be designated a hazardous product under the appropriate laws in the United States and Canada. Designating tobacco as a hazardous product would really help legislators pass the kinds of laws that can restrict smoking and cut down its appeal. This designation would allow plain packaging, larger package warnings, and allow tobacco to be taxed at the very early points of production and manufacture.

events, or other public activities. It is even suspect for tobacco companies to sponsor "anti-smoking" campaigns using their logos. Any "good" that tobacco companies do sends subliminal messages to the public—particularly to children and teenagers—that cigarettes are somehow linked to something acceptable.

Although there have been strong efforts by North American governments to limit cigarette advertising, we still see lively, colorful print ads in magazines and on billboards that promote smoking. Any kind of advertising, including sponsorship, allows tobacco companies to sport their logos. Print advertising in women's magazines continues to send seductive messages to young women, who link smoking to beauty and, most of all, to thinness. As a consumer you have the power to stop this: boycott events that are sponsored by tobacco companies, and be sure to contact the boycotted organization to let them know that they've lost you as a patron because of their willingness to use tobacco dollars.

And don't feel guilty, either! Tobacco sponsorship is unethical in all but one scenario: paying for or sponsoring treatment of smoking-related illnesses, and compensating people who are debilitated by smoking-related illnesses.

Restricting or prohibiting sponsorship may appear to punish the organizations that need the money, but we cannot afford to continue to send mixed messages. At the very least, if organizations want to continue to take "dirty money," public health and primary prevention experts suggest that governments prohibit the use of tobacco product names, trademarks, colors and logos in all tobacco-sponsorship advertising.

Removing the incentive for organizations to accept sponsorship from the tobacco industry is another way to address the problem. The state of Victoria, Australia, for example, formed the Victoria Health Promotion

Stopping Cancer at the Source

Foundation with just such an incentive in mind. Funded by tobacco taxes, the foundation's mandate is to support the sports and cultural groups that refuse tobacco industry funding. Our governments could offer a similar alternative by working with cancer and other health organizations to pool resources to provide such support, especially by using some of the revenue from tobacco taxation. And if we increase taxes on tobacco even further, the eventual return could be funneled back into the health care system, improving the quality of life for all of us.

Making Good Use of Tobacco Dollars

Billions of dollars per year are spent treating people with smoking-related illnesses. This is an enormous economic burden to place on society, especially when it is clear that *prevention is possible*. Most U.S. states have launched lawsuits against the tobacco industry. In 1998, following the publication of the *Vanity Fair* article "The Man Who Knew Too Much," lawsuits against big tobacco, filed first by Mississippi, and then by 40 other states, were eventually settled at U.S. $246 billion. Other jurisdictions have considered increased taxation on the tobacco industry as a means of seeking payback for the harm caused by the sale of its products.

In the meantime, if you have been harmed by smoking, or know someone who has, investigate litigation against tobacco companies as a possible form of compensation.

Compensation cases
Making tobacco companies pay for smoking-related illnesses is analogous to some landmark health law cases, including the case of Dow Chemical and its silicone breast implant settlement.

When women began questioning the safety of silicone implants, and more women came forward with complaints of chronic joint pains, fatigue, rheumatoid arthritis-like symptoms and a host of other ailments that were linked to breast implants, people took notice. The U.S. Food and Drug Administration (FDA) commissioner, Dr. David Kessler, imposed a temporary ban of silicone breast implants in January 1992. And Dow Corning Corporation announced that it was not only getting out of the implant business altogether, but also releasing a series of compensation packages to women. In addition to setting up a $10 million fund to monitor breast implants in North American women who'd received them, the company would pay up to $1,200 to U.S. women who could not afford surgical removal of their implants. With only about $250 million in liability insurance, Dow Corning faced more than $1 billion in lawsuits from U.S. women.

By December 1993, a jury awarded Mariann Hopkins, 48, $7.34 million in damages for breast implants she had done in 1977, which ruptured. Including this landmark award, 9,000 individual lawsuits and 41 class action suits had been filed against Dow Corning Corporation and other implant manufacturers.

In March 1994, Dow Corning, Bristol-Myers Squibb and Baxter Healthcare announced the National Breast Implant Plaintiffs' Coalition, which was a joint compensation package. This global settlement package would provide more than $4 billion to women who suffered ill health as a result of silicone breast implants. This fund would be distributed over a thirty-year period, and would cover roughly 80 percent of the estimated $4 billion settlement costs. A breast implant recipient could either reject or accept the offer, pursuing her insurance claim if she didn't like the offer. The payments depended on age and severity of medical problems. The younger the claimant, the more money would be paid out over her lifetime.

There are other stories in the "naked city" of big bad corporations being made to pay for the harms they caused. One of the most notorious compensation cases involved the manufacturers of an intrauterine device (IUD) known as the Dalkon Shield, which was banned in 1975 and recalled in 1980. This was a badly designed, untested IUD that was rushed onto the market by the pharmaceutical firm A. H. Robins Company. At this time, IUDs did not require FDA approval. A. H. Robins purchased the rights to the Dalkon Shield from physician Dr. Hugh Davis in 1970, but the pharmaceutical company didn't conduct any tests on the IUD. It relied solely on the research of Dr. Davis, which was faulty. Furthermore, since Davis was both testing and marketing the device himself, he was in violation of professional ethics.

Insertion of the Dalkon Shield was painful, and there was a very high rate of infection among users. The device was banned in 1975 as a result. By 1976, 17 deaths had been linked to its use, but Robins took no action until 1980, when it finally recalled the device, advising physicians to remove it from all users. Robins' failure to act quickly resulted in several lawsuits, and the company went bankrupt in 1985. As of that date, 10,000 lawsuits had been brought against it. By 1986, several pharmaceutical companies in the United States, who feared the same predicament, discontinued their IUD lines.

By taking some cues from the past, we may be able to end smoking

Stopping Cancer at the Source

through litigation.

Counseling Against Smoking

Health care providers are bound by professional ethics and their legal duties

---

Investigating Tobacco

The 1999 film *The Insider* documents the ugly truth about what the tobacco industry has suppressed. Since 1996, investigations and lawsuits into the clearly unethical and harmful practices of the tobacco industry revealed shocking information that showed companies:

- Suppressing evidence linking tobacco with ill health.
- Using nicotine to enhance the addictive properties of tobacco. Cigarette manufacturing, in this case, becomes all about "nicotine delivery."
- Circulating misleading information masking the health consequences of smoking.
- Using advertising that targets vulnerable groups. These ad campaigns sink to terrible lows in their intent to appeal to children, young women, and low-income individuals.
- Exporting tobacco products to developing nations, often with accompanying advertising aimed at minors or other groups who don't have the income to support a nicotine addiction.

---

of care to counsel you and your family against harmful practices that can affect your health. That includes counseling against smoking or environmental tobacco smoke.

The advice and support of a physician really can help a smoker to quit, or can even prevent someone from starting. Unfortunately, not all health care providers adequately counsel their patients about the dangers of smoking. Health care providers include all health professionals, such as nurses, pharmacists, nurse practitioners, dentists, dermatologists and community health workers. Counseling on all these levels can help in the war against tobacco.

Contact your local health department, and ask that your local government's doctors receive continuing education regarding smoking cessation and reduction of ETS; give away educational materials on ETS reduction and smoking cessation programs; and undergo special training in smoking cessation and ETS counseling, to designate them smoking cessation counselors.

WOMEN AND SMOKING

The results are in: many young women begin smoking to control their weight. Seventy-five percent of North American women believe they are overweight, even though their body weight is normal for their size, height and age. A *New York Times* poll found that 36 percent of girls aged 13–17 wanted to change their looks. A 1995 survey of girls in Grades 9 through 12 conducted by the Centers for Disease Control in the United States found that 60 percent of them were trying to lose weight, and that 5–10 percent of girls 14 and over suffer from eating disorders. In Canada, one in nine women between the ages of 14 and 25 has an eating disorder, but this is certainly an underreported problem. Not surprising, 90 percent of all eating disorders are diagnosed in women.

Tobacco ads in women's magazines continue to sell the message to young women that smoking is beautiful or glamorous. As of 1999, one brand sported the copy "It's a woman's thing," showing a beautiful, thin woman in a natural setting. Boycotting women's magazines that accept tobacco ads is one thing you, as a consumer, can do to discourage such blatantly harmful advertising. Again, it's important that your boycott or protest be followed up with a letter to the magazine's publisher and editor, explaining why you're taking this action against their publication. Tobacco companies have also sponsored fashion events and other women-related events. Once more, boycotting these events, with follow-up letters to the organizations explaining your reasons, is an important act of protest you, as a consumer, have the power to make.

Smoking and Weight Control

Many women use cigarettes as a tool for weight loss, or worse, revisit the habit long after they've quit if they are dieting. Smoking suppresses the appetite and satisfies mouth hunger—the need to have something in your mouth. But the irony is that smoking and obesity often coexist. Although some women begin to smoke in their teens as a way to lose weight, a 1997 study done by the Department of Psychology and Preventive Medicine at the University of Memphis in Tennessee shows that this approach doesn't work. Smoking teens are just as likely to become obese over time as non-smoking teens. Ironically, it was found that the more a person weighed, the more cigarettes she smoked. In the long run, smokers often wound up weighing more than non-smokers because they substituted food for nicotine when they quit or attempted to quit.

This leads not only to higher rates of smoking-related cancers, but a host of health problems linked to the catastrophic quartet: obesity; smoking; sedentary lifestyle; high blood pressure and/or high cholesterol. Smoking women also tend to go into earlier menopause, while older smokers have 20–30 percent less bone mass than non-smokers, predisposing them to bone loss and osteoporosis-linked fractures.

A CIGAR IS NOT JUST A CIGAR

Cigar smoking came back into vogue in the late 1990s. When you smoke a

---

Chinese Women and "Oil Smoke"

Chinese women worldwide are developing lung cancer in high numbers, yet few of them smoke. New research shows that oils used in cooking (such as indoor Chinese-style wok cooking, which causes the oil to smoke) can also increase the risk of lung cancer. A joint Canadian and Chinese study reported in the journal *Epidemiology*, found that Chinese women had higher rates of lung cancer because of smoking oils (rapeseed oil, in particular) used in cooking. In these cases, they were frequently stir-frying with cooking oils at high temperatures in non-separate kitchens. In general, oils, when heated to high temperatures in woks, emit potentially cancer-causing fumes. Researchers attribute higher rates of lung cancer in Chinese women who live in Shanghai, Singapore, Hong Kong, Taiwan, the United States, Australia and Malaysia to this practice. Studies show that women who stir-fried with unrefined rapeseed oil had an 84 percent increased risk of developing lung cancer, compared with women who used other types of cooking oils.

---

cigar, you're getting filler, binder and wrapper, which are made of air-cured and fermented tobaccos. Like cigarette tobacco, lit cigars emit more than four thousand chemicals, of which 43 are known to cause cancer.

Since cigars are not inhaled and are so expensive, few people are addicted, and tend to smoke them as a pastime rather than an all-the-time event. Cigar smoking is a dangerous activity nonetheless, and is still the cause of mouth and other cancers.

Cigar (and pipe) smokers have higher death rates than non-smokers for most smoking-related diseases, although they are not nearly as high as death rates in cigarette smokers. When the nicotine is absorbed through the mouth, however, cigar/pipe smokers, as well as anyone using chewing tobacco or snuff, are at higher risk of laryngeal, oral and esophageal cancer. Cigar/pipe smokers also have higher death rates than non-smokers from chronic obstructive lung disease as well as lung cancer. Heart disease is the one thing that cigar/pipe smokers are not at higher risk for than non-smokers.

Cigar smoking is a pastime that is being sold to women as something that is attractive and sexy. And women are actually buying into it, when in fact they are much more attracted to the maleness of the cigar and the "male world" it evokes for them. We need to start anti-cigar smoking campaigns to end mouth and other related cancers. Since this trend is attractive to higher-income groups, anti-cigar smoking campaigns should be targeting universities and other centers of higher learning, as well as large corporations.

QUITTING SMOKING

In order to prevent smoking-related lung cancer, which accounts for roughly 90 percent of lung cancers, and other smoking-related diseases, we can't just focus on getting people to quit smoking; we have to focus on preventing people from starting. Studies show that any real health benefits that long-term ex-smokers (that is, people who smoked from their teen years until age 55 or so) gain from quitting are not noticeable until at least fifteen years after they quit. This fact was shown in the American Cancer Society's Cancer Prevention Study, where the death rates of former smokers did not begin to match those of never-smokers until 15–20 years after the smokers quit. If you smoked for only a short period of time, or quit smoking in your thirties or forties, the health benefits will be seen much more quickly.

Smoking Cessation Programs

If you are attempting to quit smoking through some of the following smoking cessation methods, request reimbursement from your cigarette-brand manufacturer. You should also seek out other quitters who may want to launch a class action suit for recovering smoking cessation costs from tobacco manufacturers. And you may want to ask your workplace to fund a smoking cessation program, seeking funding from tobacco companies or using tobacco money the government accumulates to fund the smoking cessation program.

- Behavioral counseling: Behavioral counseling, either group or individual, can raise the rate of abstinence 20–25 percent. This approach to smoking cessation aims to change the mental processes of smoking, reinforce the benefits of non-smoking and teach skills to help the smoker avoid the urge to smoke.

- Nicotine Gum: Nicotine (Nicorette) gum is now available over the counter in Canada and the United States. It works as an aid to help you quit smoking by reducing nicotine cravings and withdrawal symptoms. Nicotine gum helps you wean yourself from nicotine by allowing you to decrease the dosage gradually until you stop using the gum altogether, a process that usually takes about 12 weeks. The only disadvantage with this method is that it caters to the oral and addictive aspects of smoking by rewarding the urge to smoke with a dose of nicotine.

- Nicotine Patch: Transdermal nicotine, or the patch (Habitrol, Nicoderm, Nicotrol), doubles abstinence rates in former smokers. Most brands are now available over the counter in both Canada and the United States. Each morning a new patch is applied to a different area of dry, clean, hairless skin and left on for the day. Some patches are designed to be worn a full 24 hours. However, the constant supply of nicotine to the bloodstream sometimes causes very vivid or disturbing dreams. You can also expect to feel a mild itching, burning or tingling at the site of the patch when it is first applied. The nicotine patch works best when it is worn for at least 7–12 weeks, with a gradual decrease in strength, that is, nicotine. Many smokers find it effective because it allows them to tackle the psychological addiction to smoking before they are forced to deal with the physical symptoms of withdrawal.

- Nicotine Inhaler: The nicotine inhaler (Nicotrol Inhaler) delivers nicotine orally via inhalation from a plastic tube. Its success rate is about 28 percent, similar to that of nicotine gum. It's available by prescription only in the United States, and has yet to make its debut in Canada. Like nicotine gum, the inhaler mimics smoking behavior by responding to each craving or urge to smoke, a feature that has both advantages and disadvantages to the smoker who wants to get over the physical symptoms of withdrawal. The nicotine inhaler should be used for a period of 12 weeks.

- Nicotine Nasal Spray: Like nicotine gum and the nicotine patch, nicotine nasal spray reduces craving and withdrawal symptoms, allowing smokers to cut back gradually. One squirt delivers about 1 mg nicotine. In three clinical trials involving 730 patients, 31–35 percent were not smoking at 6 months. This compares to an average of 12–15 percent of smokers who were able to quit unaided. The nasal spray has a couple of advantages over the gum and the patch: nicotine is rapidly absorbed across the nasal membranes, providing a kick that is more like the real thing; and the prompt onset of action plus a flexible dosing schedule benefits heavier smokers. Because the nicotine reaches your bloodstream so quickly, nasal sprays do have a greater potential for addiction than the slower-acting gum and patch. Nasal sprays are not yet available for use in Canada.

- Bupropion: Bupropion (Zyban) is appropriate for patients who have been unsuccessful using nicotine replacement. Formerly prescribed as an antidepressant, Bupropion was discovered by accident: researchers knew that smokers who were trying to quit were often depressed, and so they began experimenting with the drug as a means to fight depression, not addiction. Bupropion reduces the withdrawal symptoms associated with smoking cessation and can be used in conjunction with nicotine replacement therapy.

  Researchers suspect that Bupropion works directly in the brain to disrupt the addictive power of nicotine by affecting the same chemical neurotransmitters (or messengers) in the brain, such as dopamine, that nicotine does. The pleasurable aspect of addictive drugs like nicotine and cocaine is triggered by the release of dopamine. Smoking floods the brain with dopamine.

  The *New England Journal of Medicine* published the results of a study of more than 600 smokers taking Bupropion. At the end of treatment, 44 percent of those who took the highest dose of the drug (300 mg) were not smoking, compared with 19 percent of the group who took a placebo (a "dummy" pill). By the end of one year, 23 percent of the 300 mg group and 12 percent of the placebo group were still smoke-free. Using Zyban with nicotine replacement therapy seems to improve the quit rate a bit further. Four-week quit rates from the study were 23 percent for placebo; 36 percent for the patch; 49 percent for Zyban; and 58 percent for the combination of Zyban and the patch.

- Alternative therapies: Hypnosis, meditation and acupuncture have helped some smokers quit. In the case of hypnosis and meditation, sessions may be private or part of a group smoking cessation program.

If you grouped cancers into categories, a number of them, among them lung cancer, would be said to be linked to environmental toxins. Clearly, tobacco is the most easily preventable environmental toxin. Another group of cancers can be linked to diet, such as colon and other gastrointestinal cancers, as well as all the estrogen-dependent cancers, such as breast, prostate, ovarian and endometrial. The next chapter looks at what we can change in our diet to stop cancer at the source.

3
YOU ARE WHAT YOU EAT...AND DRINK

Why is the amount of fat on your body a factor in cancer risk? Two reasons. First, fat serves as an excellent host for fat-soluble toxins. So, by staying lean, you will house fewer toxins. Second, many cancers are estrogen-dependent, that is, the estrogen your body produces can make a cancer cell thrive. Estrogen-dependent cancers include breast, ovarian, uterine, colon and prostate cancers. Since fat cells make estrogen, the more fat on your body, the more estrogen you make.

This chapter addresses appropriate dietary changes you can make or demand with your consumer powers to reduce certain cancers. This information is written with the assumption that your food is from a safe and healthy food supply. Food contaminants are discussed in chapter 8.

Human and animal studies point to the same conclusion: diet can both increase your risk of cancer and reduce your risk. Dietary risk factors have been linked to a number of common cancers, including stomach, breast, colon and prostate. Protective factors, especially those derived from plant foods like fruits and vegetables, have been associated with reduced risk of many cancers. Most cancer experts agree that next to smoking, diet is the second leading modifiable cause of cancer. That means by modifying your diet you can reduce your risk of cancer.

LINKING CANCER TO DIET

Studies show that people who consume large amounts of dietary fat and meat are more likely to develop, and die from, breast and colon cancer, as well as cancers of the ovary, kidney, endometrium (lining of the uterus) and lung. One of the problems with ecological studies is that while they indicate trends in particular groups of people, they can't tell us how and why each individual's diet affects him or her. There are so many other factors that can affect diet, including childbearing patterns, genetics, activity levels and stress.

Studies measuring dietary links to cancer are fraught with complications. For example, it's hard for study participants to remember their food intake accurately if they're keeping journals. And since there are many components within one item (a hamburger, for example, has starches, proteins, condiment chemicals and the vegetables that garnish it), even a superb record from a study participant can be hard to analyze.

Just how much cancer is linked to poor diet? Estimates vary from 15–75 percent, but in light of more recent studies, it looks as if we're hovering at 30 percent, which is very significant. That said, based on studies to date, some cancers can absolutely be linked to diet, such as colon, ovarian and advanced prostate cancer, while the link between diet and other cancers still remains foggy, such as the link between diet and breast cancer. Within the fog, however, are some absolute facts:

1. Saturated fat (see page 55) is linked to higher rates of colon, ovarian and prostate cancers. (Red meat is associated more with colon and advanced prostate cancer.)

2. Daily consumption of fresh fruits and vegetables may reduce the risks of a number of cancers, including those of the mouth, pharynx, esophagus, stomach, colon, rectum, larynx, lung, breast and bladder.

3. Both soluble and insoluble fiber (see page 52) is good for you; experts are not entirely sure why. Is it the beneficial ingredients in high-fiber foods? Is it the regularity that fiber promotes? Right now, since all the good foods are also high in fiber, we are promoting high-fiber diets, but some experts think it's better to promote a high fruit and vegetable diet.

Diet and Colon Cancer: We Can Prove It

No expert in colon cancer will deny this fact: colon cancer can be reduced by diet. Of all the studies done on the link between cancer and dietary fat, the strongest connections can be made between high-fat diets and colon cancer. In other words, people who consume high quantities of fat have higher rates of colon cancer; people who consume low quantities of fat have lower rates of colon cancer.

As for fiber, studies show that people who consume high quantities of fiber have lower rates of colon cancer; people who consume low quantities of fiber have higher rates of colon cancer. In addition, people who have regular bowel movements have lower incidences of colon cancer than people who are chronically constipated. Studies comparing bowel habits of North Americans to Africans, for example, show that the incidence of colon cancer is higher in North Americans, who have less frequent bowel movements than Africans. Since we know what is constipating, we can learn from these studies, and modify our diets accordingly.

Studies also show that the amount of calories in your diet—regardless of whether they're from fat or fiber—can increase your risk of colon cancer. One study found that in people under 67 years old, an extra 500 calories a day can increase colon cancer risk in men by 15 percent and in women by 11 percent.

By lowering fat and increasing fiber, therefore, you'll greatly reduce your risk of colon cancer. In fact, experts believe that by following a low-fat, high-fiber diet, you may be able to avoid 90 percent of all stomach and colon cancers, and 20 percent of gallbladder, pancreatic, mouth, pharynx and esophageal cancers.

Diet and Breast Cancer: What We Can't Prove

We know that breast cancer rates are four to seven times higher in the United States than in Asia. When Asian women move to the United States, their risk doubles over a decade and they seem to acquire breast cancer at U.S. rates after several generations. We don't know what accounts for this difference. Is it diet—are we eating something we shouldn't or are Asian women eating some foods when in Asia that we should? For example, Japanese diets average roughly 15 percent calories from fat; North American diets average about 40 percent calories from fat. The traditional low-fat Japanese diet of rice, vegetables and fish is light years away from the meat and high-fat diet of North Americans.

The Japanese diet is also rich in plant estrogens (called phytoestrogens), such as tofu. Phytoestrogens act as weak estrogens, which interfere with ordinary estrogen production. And since estrogen seems to promote breast tumors, anything that interferes with estrogen should, theoretically, cut the risk. Some studies suggest that phytoestrogens may be associated with lower rates of breast cancer and less severe menopausal symptoms. Phytoestrogens are found in a variety of fruits and vegetables, including all soybean and linseed products, apples, alfalfa sprouts, split peas and spinach.

Stopping Cancer at the Source

Perhaps culture is a large piece in the puzzle (for example, you'll find fewer children, more birth control and less breastfeeding in the West as opposed to more children, less birth control and more breastfeeding in Asian cultures). Some even wonder if physical activity is a factor; Asian women are more active than their Western counterparts.

Studies on dietary fat and breast cancer have not been able to prove that high-fat diets are linked to a greater breast cancer risk, however. The fat and breast cancer issue has polarized breast cancer researchers. Some will tell you that the proof is in the geography: countries with high-fat diets simply have more breast cancer. Others will tell you that there are too many variables geographically and culturally that need to be studied before the fat theory becomes fact.

What you've probably heard most about is the U.S. Nurses' Health Study, where half of the nurses enrolled (who were followed over several years) received 44 percent of their daily calories from fat, while the other half received 23 percent of their daily calories from fat. This study was analyzed by Harvard University's Walter Willett, who concluded that the study showed no difference in breast cancer risk between the two groups. Similar studies on dietary fat found the same results.

Critics of the Nurses' Health Study argue that in order to see a difference, the "fat-cutting nurses" should have been getting no more than 15 percent of their calories from fat. Another problem with dietary fat studies is that food-frequency questionnaires are used to measure what people are eating, and these are pretty crude measurement tools. Researchers also question the timing of dietary fat in a woman's life cycle. Some wonder whether low-fat diets have greater impact on breast cancer risk in childhood and adolescence, when breasts are still forming, than in adulthood, when breasts are mature.

We may know the answers to some of these questions in the year 2010, when the results from the largest dietary fat study to date are due. The Women's Health Initiative is a U.S.$628 million health trial involving 164,000 U.S. women. It intends to test whether a low-fat diet that's high in fruits, vegetables and grains leads to lower breast cancer incidence in post-menopausal women than the typical Western diet

Finally, researchers published a 1998 report that suggested a 40 percent increased risk of breast cancer in women who consumed higher levels of transfatty acids (see page 56). The risk was highest among women who consume low levels of polyunsaturated fats and high levels of transfatty acids.

Side Benefits to Healthy Eating

Adopting a healthy diet is the key to health and well being. It not only protects you from a number of cancers, but also from many chronic diseases, including diabetes, heart disease and stroke, and may also be linked to a reduction in mood disorders (high-carbohydrate diets are linked to higher rates of depression). Evidence from the United States suggests that those who follow a healthy diet tend to be better educated, too; reasons may have to do with increased abilities to focus and concentrate as a result of good nutrition.

What is clear to all health promotion experts is that it is absurd not to recommend healthy eating since we know that at least some cancers are caused by poor dietary habits. We do have enough evidence to provide guidance on what constitutes an optimal diet; waiting for the beyond-a-shadow-of-a-doubt brand of proof may take years, and why lose years of healthy eating for proof that may never come?

Dietary Guidelines for Cancer Prevention

Whether you're following the Dietary Guidelines for Americans or Canada's Guide to Healthy Eating, here are the golden rules for good eating:

- Enjoy a variety of foods.
- Emphasize cereals, breads, other grain products and fruits and vegetables.
- Choose lower-fat dairy products, leaner meats and foods prepared with little or no fat.
- Achieve and maintain a healthy body weight by enjoying regular physical activity and healthy eating.
- Limit your intake of salt, alcohol and caffeine.

Please note that new research on the dangers of too little fat or diets too high in carbohydrates has emerged since these guidelines were developed. The emphasis now is on VARIETY. Try to eat pure foods rather than packaged; try to have some fat, some protein and some carbohydrates with each meal.

MAKING THE RIGHT CHANGES TO YOUR DIET

Stopping Cancer at the Source

What you basically need to understand about good diets versus bad diets is that people who consume less saturated fats, fewer empty calories (high-starch or high-sugar items) and more fiber are generally healthier. A low-fat, high-fiber diet will definitely reduce your risk of colon cancer, possibly reduce your risk of other cancers, and definitely reduce your risk of heart disease and diabetes.

Understanding Fiber

Fiber is the part of a plant your body can't digest; it comes in the form of both water-soluble fiber (which dissolves in water) and water-insoluble fiber (which does not dissolve in water but, instead, absorbs water). While soluble and insoluble fiber do differ, they are equally beneficial.

Soluble fiber lowers the "bad" cholesterol, or low-density lipoproteins (LDL), in your body. Experts aren't entirely sure how soluble fiber works its magic, but one popular theory is that it gets mixed into the bile the liver secretes and forms a type of gel that traps the building blocks of cholesterol, thus lowering harmful LDL levels. This action is akin to a spider web trapping smaller insects

Insoluble fiber doesn't affect cholesterol levels at all, but it does regulate bowel movements. How does it do this? As the insoluble fiber moves through the digestive tract, it absorbs water like a sponge and helps to form waste into a solid form faster, making the stools larger, softer and easier to pass. Without insoluble fiber, solid waste just gets pushed down to the colon or lower intestine as always, where it is stored and dried out until you're ready to have a bowel movement. This is exacerbated by ignoring the urge, as the colon further dehydrates the waste until it becomes harder and difficult to pass, a condition known as constipation.

Insoluble fiber will help to regulate bowel movements by speeding things along. Insoluble fiber increases the transit time by increasing colon motility and limiting the length of time dietary toxins hang around the intestinal wall. As insoluble fiber moves through the digestive tract, it absorbs available water like a sponge, and helps your stools form faster, which makes them softer and easier to pass. This is why it can dramatically decrease your risk of colon cancer.

Good sources of soluble fiber include oats or oat bran, legumes (dried beans and peas), some seeds, carrots, oranges, bananas and other fruits. Soybeans are also high in soluble fiber. Studies show that people with very high cholesterol have the most to gain by eating soybeans. Soybean is also a phytoestrogen that is believed to lower the risks of estrogen-dependent cancers, as well as lower the incidence of estrogen-loss symptoms associated with menopause.

Good sources of insoluble fiber are skins from various fruits and vegetables, seeds, leafy greens and cruciferous vegetables (cauliflower, broccoli, brussels sprouts) and wheat bran and whole grains. The problem is understanding what is truly whole grain. There is an assumption that because bread is dark or brown, it's more nutritious; this isn't so. In fact, many brown breads are simply enriched white breads dyed with molasses. ("Enriched" means that nutrients lost during processing have been replaced.) High-fiber pita breads and bagels are available, but you have to search for them. A good rule is to simply look for the phrase "whole wheat" on the product label, which means that the wheat is, indeed, whole.

What's in a grain?

Most of us turn to grains and cereals to boost our fiber intake, which experts recommend should be at about 25–35 grams per day. Use the chart below to help gauge whether you're getting enough. The list measures the amount of insoluble fiber. An easy way to boost your fiber intake is to add pure wheat bran to your foods, which is available in health food stores or supermarkets in a sort of "sawdust" format. Three tablespoons of wheat bran is equal to 4.4 grams of fiber. Sprinkle 1–2 tablespoons onto cereals, rice, pasta or meat dishes. You can also sprinkle it into orange juice or low-fat yogurt. It has virtually no calories. It's important to drink a glass of water with your wheat bran, as well as a glass of water after you've finished your wheat bran-enriched meal.

Water and fiber

How many people do you know who say: "But I do eat tons of fiber and I'm still constipated!" Probably quite a few. The reason they remain constipated in spite of their high-fiber diet is that they are not drinking water with fiber. It is important to note that water means water. Milk, coffee, tea, soft drinks or juice are not a substitute for water. Unless you drink water with your fiber, the fiber will not bulk up in your colon to create the nice, soft bowel movements you desire. Think of fiber as a sponge. You must soak a dry sponge with water in order for it to be useful. Same thing here. Fiber without water is as useful as a dry sponge. *You gotta soak your fiber!* So here is the fiber/water recipe:

- Drink three glasses of water with your fiber. This means having a glass of water with whatever you're eating. Even if what you're eating does not contain much fiber, drinking water with your meal is a good habit to get into.

- Drink two glasses of water after you eat.

There are, of course, other reasons to drink lots of water throughout the day. For example, some studies show that dehydration can lead to mood swings and depression. Women are often advised by numerous health and beauty experts to drink 8–10 glasses of water per day for other reasons. Water helps you to lose weight and to have well-hydrated, beautiful skin; and it helps you to urinate regularly, important for bladder function (women, in particular, suffer from bladder infections and urinary incontinence). By drinking water with your fiber, you'll be able to get up to that 8 glasses of water per day in no time.

Understanding Fat

Fat is technically known as fatty acids, which are crucial nutrients for our cells. We cannot live without fatty acids. If you looked at each fat molecule carefully, you'd find three different kinds of fatty acids on it: saturated (solid), monounsaturated (less solid, with the exception of olive and peanut oils) and polyunsaturated (liquid) fatty acids. (When you see the term "unsaturated fat," this refers to either monounsaturated or polyunsaturated fats.)

These three fatty acids combine with glycerol to make what's chemically known as triglycerides. Each fat molecule is a link chain made up of glycerol, carbon atoms and hydrogen atoms. The more hydrogen atoms that are on that chain, the more saturated or solid the fat. The liver breaks down fat molecules by secreting bile, stored in the gallbladder, its sole function. The liver also makes cholesterol. Too much saturated fat may cause your liver to overproduce cholesterol, while the triglycerides in your bloodstream will rise, perpetuating the problem.

Fat is a good thing in moderation. But like all good things, most of us want too much of it. Excess dietary fat is by far the most damaging element in the Western diet. A gram of dietary fat contains twice the calories as the same amount of protein or carbohydrate. Fat in the diet comes from meats, dairy products and vegetable oils. Other sources of fat include coconuts (60 percent fat), peanuts (78 percent fat) and avocados (82 percent fat).

To cut through all this big fat jargon, you can boil down fat into two categories: "harmful fats" and "helpful fats," which the popular press often defines as "good fats" and "bad fats."

Harmful fats

The following are harmful fats because they can increase your risk of cardiovascular problems as well as many cancers, including colon and breast cancers. These are fats that are fine in moderation, but harmful in excess (and harmless if not eaten at all):

- *Saturated fats.* These are solid at room temperature and stimulate cholesterol production in your body when the liver has to work hard to break them down. In fact, the way that saturated fat looks prior to ingesting it is the way cholesterol will look when it lines your arteries. Foods high in saturated fat include processed meat, fatty meat, lard, butter, solid vegetable shortening, chocolate and tropical oils (coconut oil is more than 90 percent saturated). Saturated fat should be consumed only in very low amounts.
- *Trans-fatty acids.* These are factory-made fats that behave just like saturated fat in your body, often found in margarine.

Helpful fats

These are fats that are beneficial to your health, and actually protect against certain health problems. You are encouraged to use more rather than less of these fats in your diet. In fact, nutritionists suggest that you substitute harmful fats with these:

- Unsaturated fat. This kind of fat is partially solid or liquid at room temperature. The more liquid the fat, the more unsaturated it is, which, in fact, lowers your cholesterol levels. This group of fats includes monounsaturated fats and polyunsaturated fats. Sources of unsaturated fats include vegetable oils (canola, safflower, sunflower, corn) and seeds and nuts. Unsaturated fats come from plants, with the exception of tropical oils, such as coconut, which are saturated.
- Fish fats (a.k.a. omega-3 fatty acids). The fats naturally present in fish that swim in cold waters, known as omega-3 fatty acids or fish oils, are all polyunsaturated. Again, polyunsaturated fats are good for you: they lower cholesterol levels, are crucial for brain tissue and protect against heart disease. Include cold-water fish like mackerel, albacore tuna, salmon and sardines in your diet.

Factory-made fats

An assortment of factory-made fats have been introduced into our diet courtesy of food producers who are trying to give us the taste of fat without all the calories of saturated fats. Unfortunately, manufactured fats offer their own bag of horrors. That's because when a fat is made in a factory, it becomes a trans-fatty acid, a harmful fat that not only raises the level of "bad" cholesterol (LDL, or low-density lipoproteins) in your bloodstream, but also lowers the amount of "good" cholesterol (HDL, or high-density lipoproteins) that's already there.

How exactly does a trans-fatty acid come into being? Trans-fatty acids are what you get when you make a liquid oil, such as corn oil, into a more solid or spreadable substance, such as margarine. Trans-fatty acids, you might say, are the road to hell, paved with good intentions. Someone way back when thought that if you could take the "good fat"—unsaturated fat— and solidify it so it could double as butter or lard, you could eat the same things without missing the spreadable fat. That sounds like a great idea. Unfortunately, to make an unsaturated liquid fat more solid, hydrogen is added to its molecules. This process, known as hydrogenation, converts liquid fat to semi-solid fat. That ever-popular chocolate bar ingredient "hydrogenated palm oil" is a classic example of a trans-fatty acid. Hydrogenation also prolongs the shelf life of a fat, such as a polyunsaturated fat, which can oxidize when exposed to air, causing rancid odors or flavors. Deep-frying oils used in the restaurant trade are generally hydrogenated.

Trans-fatty acid is sold as a polyunsaturated or monounsaturated fat with a label that reads: "Made from polyunsaturated vegetable oil." Except in your body, it is treated as a saturated fat. So, really, trans-fatty acids are a saturated fat in disguise. The advertiser may, in fact, say that the product contains "no saturated fat" or is "healthier" than the comparable animal or tropical oil product with saturated fat. So be careful out there: read your labels. The magic word you're looking for is "hydrogenated." If the product lists a variety of unsaturated fats (monounsaturated X oil, polyunsaturated Y oil), keep reading. If the word "hydrogenated" appears, count that product as a saturated fat; your body will!

Since the news of trans-fatty acids broke in the late 1980s, margarine manufacturers began to offer some less "bitter" margarines; some contain no hydrogenated oils, while others have much smaller amounts. Margarines with less than 60–80 percent oil (9 to 11 grams of fat) will contain 1 to 3 grams of trans-fatty acids per serving, compared to butter, which is 53 percent saturated fat. You might say it's a choice between a bad fat and a worse fat.

It's also possible for a liquid vegetable oil to retain a high concentration of unsaturated fat when it's been partially hydrogenated. In this case, your body will metabolize this as some saturated fat and some unsaturated fat.

Fake fat

We have artificial sweeteners; why not artificial fat? This question has led to the creation of a highly suspicious ingredient: fat substitutes, designed to replace real fat and hence reduce the calories and dangers from real fat without compromising the taste. This is done by creating a fake fat that the body cannot absorb.

One of the first fat substitutes was Simplesse, an "All-Natural Fat Substitute," made from milk and egg-white protein, which was developed by the NutraSweet Company. Simplesse apparently adds 1–2 calories per gram instead of the usual 9 calories per gram from fat. Other fat substitutes simply take protein and carbohydrates and modify them in some way to simulate the textures of fat (creamy, smooth, etc.). All of these fat substitutes help to create low-fat products.

The calorie-free fat substitute promoted recently is called Olestra, developed by Procter & Gamble. Olestra is a potentially dangerous ingredient that most experts believe can do more harm than good. The product is currently being test marketed in the United States in a variety of savory snacks, such as potato chips and crackers. Canada has not yet approved it.

Olestra is made from a combination of vegetable oils and sugar. Therefore, it tastes just like the real thing, but the biochemical structure is a molecule too big for your liver to break down. So, Olestra just gets passed into the large intestine and is excreted. Olestra is more than an "empty" molecule, however. According to the U.S. Commissioner of Food and Drugs, Olestra may cause diarrhea and cramps and may deplete the body of vital nutrients, including vitamins A, D, E and K, necessary for blood to clot. Indeed, all studies conducted by Procter & Gamble have shown this potential. If the FDA approves Olestra for use as a cooking-oil substitute, you'll see it in every imaginable high-fat product. In a critique of Olestra published in a 1996 issue of the *University of California at Berkeley Wellness Letter* (the year Olestra was approved for test markets), nutritionists suggested that instead of encouraging people to choose nutritious foods, such as fruits, grains and vegetables over high-fat foods, products like Olestra encourage a high fake-fat diet that's still too low in fiber and other essential nutrients. Products like Olestra should make you nervous.

Understanding Carbohydrates

Stopping Cancer at the Source

Fat is not the only thing that can make you fat. A diet high in carbohydrates can also make you fat. That's because carbohydrates (starchy stuff, such as rice, pasta, breads or potatoes) can be stored as fat when eaten in excess. Carbohydrates can be simple or complex. Simple carbohydrates are found in any food that contains natural sugar (honey, fruits, juices, vegetables, milk) and anything that contains table sugar. Complex carbohydrates are more sophisticated foods that are made up of larger molecules, such as grain foods, starches and foods high in fiber.

Normally, all carbs convert into glucose when you eat them. Glucose is the technical term for "simplest sugar." All your energy comes from the glucose in your blood, also known as blood glucose or blood sugar. When your blood sugar is used up, you feel weak, tired and hungry. But what happens when you eat more carbohydrates than your body can use? Your body stores those extra carbs as fat. What we also know is that the rate at which glucose is absorbed by your body from carbohydrates is affected by other parts of your meal, such as the protein, fiber and fat you consume. If you're eating only carbohydrates and no protein or fat, for example, they will convert into glucose more quickly, to the point where you may experience mood swings as your blood sugar rises and dips.

Nutritionists advise that each meal should contain roughly 50–55 percent carbohydrates, 15–20 percent protein, and less than 30 percent fat.

Understanding Sugar

Sugars are found naturally in many of the foods you eat. The simplest form of sugar is glucose, your basic body fuel. You can buy pure glucose at any drugstore in the form of dextrose tablets. Dextrose is just "edible glucose." When people are fed "sugar water" intravenously, dextrose is the sugar in that water. When you see the word "dextrose" on a candy-bar label, it means that the manufacturer used edible glucose in the recipe. Glucose is the baseline ingredient of all naturally occurring sugars, which include:

- Sucrose: table or white sugar, naturally found in sugar cane and sugar beets.
- Fructose: the natural sugar in fruits and vegetables.
- Lactose: the natural sugar in all milk products.
- Maltose: the natural sugar in grains (flours and cereals).

When you ingest a natural sugar of any kind, you're actually ingesting one part glucose and one or two parts of another naturally occurring sugar. For example, sucrose is biochemically constructed from one part glucose and one part fructose. So, from glucose it came, and unto glucose it shall return, once it hits your digestive system. The same is true for all naturally occurring sugars, with the exception of lactose. As it happens, lactose breaks down into glucose and an "odd duck" simple sugar, galactose.

How long does it take for one of the above sugars to return to glucose? Well, it greatly depends on the amount of fiber in your food, how much protein you've eaten and how much fat accompanies the sugar in your meal. Again, if you have enough energy or fuel, once that sugar becomes glucose, it can be stored as fat. And that's how—and why—sugar can make you fat.

Factory-added sugars
You also have to watch out for added sugars; these are sugars that manufacturers add to foods during processing or packaging. Foods containing fruit juice concentrates, invert sugar, regular corn syrup, honey or molasses and hydrolyzed lactose syrup or high-fructose corn syrup (made out of highly concentrated fructose through the hydrolysis of starch) contain added sugars.

Many people don't realize, however, that pure, unsweetened fruit juice is still a potent source of sugar, even when it contains no added sugar. Extra lactose, dextrose and maltose are also contained in many of your foods. In other words, the products may have naturally occurring sugars anyway, and then more sugar is thrown in to enhance consistency and taste. The best way to know how much sugar a product contains is to look at the nutritional label for "carbohydrates."

WHO CAN HELP US EAT BETTER?

Knowing all the fiber/fat/sugar information is not going to help you eat well if you don't have access to a healthy, high-quality food supply or food labels you can read and understand. So what can we do as consumers to help business and government make it easier for us?

When we think about who protects our diet we may look to departments or ministries of health, food, water, agriculture, finance, education, industry, social services and trade. Agrifood departments or ministries are certainly the most important players in our diet, but don't forget that they have to work together with food retailers and food services to help promote high-quality foods, healthy eating habits and, most important, access to a healthy food supply. By looking at the way food is produced, stored and distributed, policies can be introduced by government and industry to help ensure that good food is available to all of us.

Getting the Food Industry on Our Side

Ideally, we want those in the food industry responsible for the production of fruit, vegetables and high-fiber grain products, as well as the producers and distributors of lower-fat meat and dairy products, to get more of their foods on food retailers' shelves. You may have tried to "healthy food-shop" in smaller cities or towns and noticed the absence of fresh foods, or the absence of variety in "outside aisles." This is a food industry and food distribution problem. The first thing you can do is contact your local food retailers and ask them where they buy their produce so you can locate the right channels to voice your concerns.

You may also notice that you can buy seven different kinds of brand-name cereals, but can't find a bag of natural oats or generic natural grain cereals. Again, this is a food industry problem, where brand-name, more expensive and less nutritious products are often shelved because the profit margins are higher. In these cases, you can contact the food industry and make your demands known for more variety in products, particularly generic alternatives to brand names. Since the food industry is very concerned with what consumers want, they are more apt to respond to consumer demands.

Food Labels

Surveys continuously reveal that shoppers consider nutrition to be either very important or extremely important. They also reveal that consumers rely on packages and labels for nutrition information, but that in most cases, find the ingredients list of certain products—especially processed and artificial food products—hard to decipher. In cases where food products are designed to mimic or substitute natural favorites like cheese, meat and fish, consumers find assessing nutritional value difficult. We need labels that everyone can understand. In cases where it would be cumbersome to attach a label containing nutritional information to a food product (for example, a cinnamon bun baked in the store), the nutritional breakdown could be provided by the cashier at point-of-purchase.

So who's responsible for our food labels? The state departments/ ministries of health, agriculture, food and rural affairs are chiefly responsible for developing nutritional labeling systems. If you're not happy with food labels, contacting these departments/ministries, as well as the product manufacturers, can help to bring about changes in the way nutritional information is presented.

Making sense of labels

Nutritional information on food labels must make sense. It's not enough that labels are written in plain English; they need to address the dietary concerns of consumers.

For example, since 1993 in the United States, food labels have been adhering to strict guidelines set out by the Food and Drug Administration (FDA) and the U.S. Department of Agriculture's (USDA) Food Safety and Inspection Service (FSIS). All labels will list "Nutrition Facts" on the side or back of the package. The " % Daily Values" column tells you how high or low that food is in various nutrients, such as fat, saturated fat, and cholesterol. A number of 5 or less is "low"—good news if the product shows <5 for fat, saturated fat, and cholesterol—bad news if the product is <5 for fiber. Serving sizes are also confusing. Foods that are similar are given the same type of serving size defined by the FDA. That means that 5 cereals that all weigh X grams per cup will share the same serving sizes.

Calories (how much energy) and calories from fat (how much fat) are also listed per serving of food. Total carbohydrate, dietary fiber, sugars, other carbohydrates (i.e., starches), total fat, saturated fat, cholesterol, sodium, potassium and vitamins and minerals are given in Percent Daily values, based on the 2,000-calorie diet recommended by the U.S. government. (In Canada, Recommended Nutrient Intake (RNI) is used for vitamins and minerals, while ingredients on labels are listed according to weight, with the "most" listed first.)

But that's not where the confusion ends—or even begins! You have to wade through the various "claims" and understand what they mean. For example anything that is "X-free" (as in sugar-free, saturated fat-free, cholesterol-free, sodium-free, calorie-free and so on) means that the product indeed has "no X" or that "X" is so tiny, it is dietarily insignificant. This is not the same thing as a label that says "95% fat-free." In this case, the product contains relatively small amounts of fat, but still has fat. This claim is based on 100 grams of the product. For example, if a snack food contains 2.5 grams of fat per 50 grams, it can be said to be "95% fat-free."

A label that screams "low in saturated fat"or "low in calories" is not fat-free or calorie-free. It means that you can eat a large amount of that food without exceeding the Daily Value for that food. In potato-chip country, that could mean you can eat 12 potato chips instead of 6. So if you eat the whole bag of "low-fat" chips, you're still eating a lot of fat. Be sure to check serving sizes.

"Cholesterol-free" or "low cholesterol" means that the product doesn't have any, or much, animal fat (hence, cholesterol). This doesn't mean "low fat." Pure vegetable oil doesn't come from animals but is pure fat!

And then there are the "comparison claims" such as "fewer," "reduced," "less," "more," or my favorite—"light" (or worse, "lite"). These words appear on foods that have been nutritionally altered from a previous version or competitor's version. For example, Regular Brand X Potato Chips may have much more fat than Lite Brand X Potato Chips "with less fat than Regular Brand X." That doesn't mean that Lite Brand X is fat-free or even low in fat. It just means it's *lower* in fat than Regular Brand X.

On the flip side, Brand Y may have a trace amount of calcium, while Brand Y "now with more calcium" may still have a small amount of calcium, but 10% more than Brand Y. (In other words, you may still need to eat 100 bowls of Brand Y before you get the daily requirement for calcium!)

To be light or "lite"a product has to contain either one-third fewer calories or half the fat of the regular product. Or, a low-calorie or low-fat food contains 50% less sodium. Something that is "light in sodium" means it has at least 50% less sodium than the regular product, such as canned soup. (But if you're buying hair color that reads "light brown," it is a descriptive word only, you can be sure!)

When a label says sugar-free, it contains less than 0.5 grams of sugar per serving, while a "reduced-sugar" food contains at least 25 percent less sugar per serving than the regular product. If the label also states that the product is not a reduced or low-calorie food, or it is not for weight control, it's got enough sugar in there to make you think twice. But sugar-free in the language of labels simply means sucrose-free. That doesn't mean the product is carbohydrate-free, as in: dextrose-free, lactose-free, glucose-free or fructose-free. Check the labels for all things ending in "ose" to find out the sugar content; you're not just looking for sucrose. Watch out for "no added sugar," "without added sugar" or "no sugar added." This simply means: "We didn't put the sugar in, God did." Again, reading the number of carbohydrates on the nutrition information label is the most accurate way to know the amount of sugar in the product.

The Problem of Poverty

Poverty is an enormous barrier to a healthy diet and lifestyle, and while the problem used to be particularly rampant in the seniors' community, it is now more of a problem in single mother-led families.

Because they may not have the money to spend on transportation, many low-income families shop for food at small convenience stores where the quality and selection of healthy food products, such as fresh vegetables, are limited. Ironically, convenience store prices are generally higher than those at suburban grocery stores. Transportation barriers also exist for the disabled, which, again, limit grocery shopping locations. And since poverty and poor literacy skills often go hand in hand, complicated nutrition labels

Commonly Used U.S. and Canadian Nutrient Claim Comparisons

Claim	U.S.	Canada
"Low Calorie"	40 calories or less per serving.	50 percent less energy than a regular product and 15 calories or less per serving.
"Low Fat"	3 grams of fat or less per serving.	3 grams of fat or less per serving
"Low Cholesterol"	20 mg of cholesterol or less per serving (in addition to saturated fat and total fat restrictions)	20 mg of cholesterol or less per serving (in addition to the saturated fat restrictions only)

can be a real barrier to accessing healthy foods.

If you're struggling to put nutritious food on the table, there are things you can do to help put more nutritious foods into your local grocery store:

- Together with others in your community who share the same problem, look into alternative methods of shopping or eating through community kitchens, food-buying clubs and networking with farmers, who may be willing to do "field-to-table programs." You could also start a community garden.
- Contact food manufacturers and encourage them to donate all unused fresh produce and other healthy foods to food banks or community kitchens.
- If you're a parent, get your school board to institute a school breakfast and/or lunch program to help children in need eat more nutritiously.
- Contact your city planning department and let them know that your community is in need of good food stores rather than convenience stores.

- In economically strapped communities, it might be worthwhile to contact some of the larger food stores with good selections and encourage them to invest in your community by buying out some of the deadwood retailers (such as pawnshops or money marts) and open some new stores. This trend is seen in many large urban centers as part of urban renewal programs.

Marketing Board and Producer Associations

State and provincial marketing boards and producer associations that work with our farmers are an important part of the food production and distribution system. Most of these boards and associations are involved in the quality production of fruits, vegetables and grains. In the last few years, in response to consumer demand for lower-fat products, the meat and dairy industries in particular are making lower-fat products available. There are also a variety of soy manufacturers who are delivering meat and dairy substitutes in the form of tofu burgers, tofu cheeses or even tofu turkeys.

Understanding grading of meat is another problem. For example, in Canada, consumers believe that the highest-quality grades (AAA) are the healthiest, when in fact they are often the fattiest. To meet AAA criteria, meat has to contain greater marbling (visible fat). Beef with no visible fat is graded B; but it may in fact be leaner. "High-quality" beef must therefore revert to its previous status as a high-fat-containing food that could prove harmful to health. So when shopping for meat, be sure to check with your local meat marketing board what your meat grading refers to.

Other Barriers to Healthy Eating

Familiarity with cooking various foods is a huge factor in buying habits. Many people are limited in their tofu or vegetarian recipes, for example, so they tend to buy foods they feel more comfortable preparing. There are also good foods that are only bad when they are cooked in oil or fat; potato wedges heated in an oven, for example, have a much lower fat content than french fries prepared in a conventional deep fryer.

Another major barrier to healthy eating is food in the workplace. All community institutions (schools, hospitals) and workplaces with a food services or vending machine should be required to provide healthy food alternatives. Nutritional information about available foods should be posted on the premises, close to where the foods are serviced. One way of enforcing this measure is to demand that nutritional requirements and ingredients lists become part of all catering contracts.

Other ways to overcome barriers to healthy eating include:

- Food skills. If you're in the know with respect to food preparation and nutritional cooking, why not volunteer this skill to your community in exchange for something else through the well-known barter system? For example, you go shopping with your neighbor; she'll make you some curtains, or he'll fix your roof. Many North Americans know very little about the principles of healthy food preparation, a phenomenon partly due to the increased popularity of fast-food outlets and microwaveable food products. They need to be educated. We need healthy-food education programs, which could be made available at the community level.

- Healthy food education campaigns. Educational initiatives (print and media campaigns) that aim to get us healthy need to be written in plain, easy-to-understand language (a Grade 6 reading level). Special efforts should also be made to convey nutritional information to people with low literacy levels. Educational initiatives encouraging better nutrition need to provide alternatives that work within a variety of cultural settings. Where numbers warrant, educational materials and/or healthy-food preparation workshops should be geared towards the different cultural preferences of the community. Contact your community organizations and suggest this initiative.

- Food education in schools. We have sex education; why not food education? Suggest this to your school board, which can collaborate with the Department/Ministry of Health and the Department/Ministry of Education to make nutrition education a necessary part of comprehensive school health programs. Our children are being bombarded with commercials on TV that sell them sugar and high-fat snack foods.

- No-junk-food in schools. Get some parents together and demand your school be a junk-food-free zone. (If schools can ban Pokéman, they can ban junk food!) The prevalence of foods low in nutritional value and/or high in fat in school cafeterias and vending machines helps to keep our children unhealthy.

- Limit sugar shows. Limit your child's access to television programming for children that is basically a vehicle to sell sugar cereals and junk food. Some foods aimed at children contain as much as 22 grams of fat and 1,500 mg of sodium. (Add in the pudding cup and you can well imagine the damage!) Selling pies and cakes as breakfast foods to children raises some ethical questions as well in that it can be argued that junk food for breakfast is harmful.

CONTROLLING ALCOHOL, PREVENTING ALCOHOLISM

It seems as though one contradictory study after another comes out about alcohol consumption and its link to various kinds of cancer. Alcohol abuse and alcoholism is one of the most common social problems of the past two centuries; but alcohol, in moderation, isn't a bad thing, and even has some health benefits.

One of the most infamous public health failures was Prohibition, which, in the United States, banned the manufacture, sale and distribution of alcohol. This is also known as the Eighteenth Amendment to the U.S. Constitution (or the Volstead Act), which passed after World War I in response to extreme conservatism.

Prohibition dominated North American life throughout the early part

---

Avoid Ruining the Right Foods

The American Institute for Cancer Research's Diet and Cancer Project, Food Nutrition and the Prevention of Cancer, recommends that by avoiding the following, you'll decrease your risk of cancer:

Avoid salted foods and table salt whenever possible; season your foods with herbs.

Avoid eating food that was "left out" for long periods of time; the food can become contaminated with bacteria.

Avoid eating perishable foods that were not refrigerated.

Avoid unlabelled foods when travelling in undeveloped or developing countries, as contaminants, additives and other residues are not properly regulated in these areas.

Avoid charred food, or meat and fish cooked over an open flame.

Avoid cured or smoked meats. The nitrites these foods contain are carcinogenic.

---

of the twentieth century (some of our grandparents may still remember it). Canada also passed prohibition laws in this same period. What we learned about Prohibition is that it didn't work, and led to unparalleled drinking of inferior and cruder alcohol concoctions that people made themselves, called bootleg. In fact, more time and energy was wasted trying to control alcohol smuggling or bootlegging, and other crimes associated with smuggling, using up law enforcement resources that should have been available for more serious problems. The enormous failure of Prohibition led to its repeal, or the Twenty-first Amendment of the U.S. Constitution in 1933; most Canadian provinces with similar laws had repealed them by this time.

In light of the lessons learned from Prohibition, why do we still want to control alcohol? Well, we still need to prevent moderate drinking from spilling over into heavy, addictive drinking, or alcoholism, which causes a number of serious health problems, including certain cancers. Approximately 10 percent of cancer deaths are at least in part attributable to alcohol. Alcohol has been identified as a cause of oral, pharynx, larynx and esophogeal cancers, especially in those who also smoke. In fact, the life-time risk of being diagnosed with these cancers is 35 times higher in people who both smoke and drink. Alcohol is also a cause of primary liver cancer (common in the aboriginal population), and a possible cause of breast and colorectal cancers. The cancers caused by alcohol are largely preventable, as are the other adverse health, social and economic consequences of heavy drinking.

One of the problems with lowering alcohol consumption is conflicting information about alcohol—especially since there is good evidence to support that alcohol can help to lower cholesterol. For example, it's also been shown that 1–2 glasses of wine daily for men and 1–3 alcoholic beverages per week for women may lower the risk of heart disease. The alcohol raises your HDL, or "good" cholesterol, thus reducing the deposits of cholesterol in the arterial walls.

So what are the official guidelines for consuming alcohol? The former Addiction Research Foundation in Toronto recommended that people who drink limit their consumption of alcoholic beverages to not more than two standard-size drinks daily, with a limit of 12 drinks weekly. (A standard-size drink or its equivalent is 1 1/2 oz. of 40 % strength liquor, 12 oz. of 5 % strength beer or 5 oz. of 12% strength wine.) Those with lower than average body weight, or those at significant risk for certain diseases or conditions, should drink less. These guidelines were created on the basis of research indicating that alcohol-related problems increase with consumption levels. When your consumption levels exceed the recommended limits, your risk factor of alcohol-related diseases is higher than it should be, too. While moderate alcohol consumption might have potential health benefits, for some cancers there may be no safe level of consumption.

Breast Cancer and Alcohol

Since much of the information on alcohol and health is based on studies of men, women are often confused about the link between cancer risk and their alcohol consumption. Using breast cancer risk rules is a good guideline for any estrogen-dependent cancer. The former Addiction Research Foundation found that 199 deaths from breast cancer in 1994 were attributable to alcohol. A woman's risk of getting breast cancer is increased by 10 percent with excessive alcohol consumption. A 1993 National Institute of Health (NIH) study found that two alcoholic drinks per day could raise a woman's estrogen levels enough to increase her risk of breast cancer by 40–100 percent over women who do not drink at all. In this study, 34 women had their blood levels checked mid-cycle, and were found to have a 31.9 percent increase in estrogen over women who were not drinking.

Preventing Alcohol Abuse

Studies have consistently shown that alcohol education aimed at our entire population can reduce the proportion of heavy drinkers and alcohol-related problems. Drinking is, after all, a social activity for many of us. By targeting the entire population with alcohol-consumption education, we can reach anyone vulnerable to alcohol abuse, a problem that is not income-specific. Alcohol abuse spans everything from drinking and driving and binge drinking (common on university campuses, for example) to full-blown alcoholism.

Liquor control boards
It's long been known that corner liquor stores in large U.S. cities help to breed alcohol abuse. This is one reason why many provinces in Canada have set up controlled distribution and sale of alcohol. Ontario is an example of a monopoly system of alcohol distribution, which has been a proven deterrent to alcohol-related problems. Ontario's current monopoly system, for example, controls the sale of a large share of alcoholic beverages in provincially run outlets—Liquor Control Board of Ontario stores (LCBOs)—and only licenses establishments that conform with LCBO regulations. Resisting leniency in advertising will be the challenge; certain alcohol-containing products, such as "coolers," are undergoing active promotion because they don't fall into any specific, controlled category, as is the case with beer, wine and hard liquor.

The best plan of action is for consumers to fight to keep existing monopolies on alcohol, or fight to create Ontario-like monopolies. Although the trend is toward the deregulation of alcohol sales, as seen in some Canadian provinces and in New Zealand, this is not a great plan. Proposals that erode current control on alcohol should be resisted if we want to keep consumption levels down.

Controlling access to alcohol, studies show, really helps reduce consumption. Legislation governing the advertising and promotion of alcoholic beverages, legal drinking age, hours of operation and retail sales, as well as the number of stores allowed per capita, are good initiatives that Ontario and other Canadian provinces follow; more U.S. cities should follow the Canadian example.

TIPS and SIPs—Training the Alcohol Servers

Properly training and educating the servers of alcohol, that is, the staff of licensed bars and restaurants, leads to fewer alcohol-related problems. This training is known as Training for Intervention Procedures (TIPS) in the United States, and Server Intervention Programs (SIPs) in Canada and involves education about the dangers of excessive drinking, including automobile accidents and violence. TIPS/SIPs help to promote and reinforce moderate drinking as the social norm, and heavy drinking as a social harm.

One of the best ways consumers can support TIPS/SIPs is to ask their favorite establishments if their staff is TIP or SIP-trained. If not, suggest this training to the owner of the establishment. It could reduce the amount of drunk drivers in your area, for example, not to mention lower the health risks associated with alcohol abuse.

TIPS/SIPs should become requirements before a liquor license is either obtained or extended.

Teaching Children about Alcohol Abuse

Not all young people wait until their legal drinking age to experiment with alcohol. The evidence shows, however, that school-based education programs delay the onset of regular drinking. The best plan is to make alcohol education part of nutrition education (see page 65) and anti-smoking education (see chapter 10). The best time to do this is during the transitional year between grade school and secondary school, when the contemplation of bad habits begins, often because of peer pressure.

We know from a myriad of good studies that lowering our fat intake and increasing our fiber intake is only one-half of whole-body health. We have to use our bodies in order to use up our calories, stay healthy and increase oxygen flow to all our cells. People who are active appear to have a lower cancer risk than those who are inactive. Sedentary living breeds ill health and a number of ailments; physical activity is one of the most important primary prevention tools in reducing cancer incidence. Chapter 4 gives you the information and incentives you'll need to get physical.

4
ACTIVE LIVING

The American and Canadian Cancer societies state that people who are active have lower rates of cancer. Active people also tend to consume more of the scarce micronutrients our bodies crave. Both of these factors have recently been associated with a reduced risk of cancer. There is evidence that even moderate amounts of physical activity will help to reduce the incidence of breast and other cancers. The 1999 Report of the Ontario Expert Panel on Colorectal Cancer Screening, the most recently published task force report in North America on strategies to prevent colon cancer, also cites physical inactivity as a chief risk factor for colon cancer.

This chapter explains how exercise can benefit you, and suggests ways to get started. It is not intended as a workout program, however. Anybody reading this chapter needs to design a doable exercise program that is appealing and convenient; for most people, that will mean combining some kind of simple stretching routine with some aerobic activity. As one expert aptly put it on her video, the program you can do is the one you will do.

People who have been sedentary most of their lives tend to be intimidated by health and fitness clubs. Walking into a room with complicated-looking machines, filled with young, fit, supple bodies is not exactly an inviting atmosphere for somebody who doesn't understand how to program a StairMaster. And the "language" of exercise is intimidating, too. Not only do you need an anatomy lesson to understand which movements stretch which group of muscles, but you need to take a crash course in cardiology to understand exactly how long you have to have your pulse at X beats per minute, with the sweat pouring off of you, before you burn any fat. The concept of "gaining muscle" over existing fat is also a hard one to grasp. While you're burning fat, you will be building some muscle—muscle weighs more than fat—so forget about weight loss and think about fat loss. And don't think you're going to end up looking like a body builder; while your muscles will become more firm or better defined, your workouts will never be as intense as a body builder's.

Aerobics classes are another problem; many people (like me) are uncomfortable with their lack of finesse in public. Moreover, many aerobics classes assume that you've had formal ballet training; after all, you need the grace of a dancer to perform half the moves! So let me stress something before you read on: you're wearing all the equipment you will ever need to exercise. If you can breathe, stretch and walk, you can become a lean mean exercise machine without paying a membership fee.

WHAT DOES EXERCISE REALLY MEAN?

Exercise has been defined as "the exertion of muscles, limbs, etc., especially for health's sake; bodily, mental or spiritual training." In the Western world, we have placed an emphasis on "bodily training" when we talk about exercise, ignoring mental and spiritual training. Only recently have Western studies begun to focus on the mental benefits of exercise. It's been shown, for example, that exercise stimulates the production of endorphins, neurotransmitters that occur naturally in the brain and make us feel good. But we in the West do not encourage meditation or other calming forms of mental and spiritual exercise, which have also been shown to improve well-being and health.

In the East, for thousands of years, exercise has focused on achieving mental and spiritual health through the body, using breathing and postures.

The Meaning of Aerobic

If you look up the word "aerobic" in the dictionary, what you'll likely find is the biochemical definition: "living in free oxygen." This is certainly correct; we are all aerobes—beings that require oxygen to live. Some bacteria are anaerobic; that is, they can exist in an environment without oxygen. All that jumping around and fast movement we engage in when we exercise is done to create faster breathing so we can take more oxygen into our bodies. Since the blood contains oxygen, the faster your blood flows, the more oxygen can flow to your organs. However, it is important to note that when your health care practitioner tells you to "exercise" or to take up "aerobic exercise," he or she is not referring solely to "increasing oxygen" but to exercising the heart muscle. The faster your heart beats, the better a workout it gets (although you don't want to overwork your heart, either). You want to make it stronger—a fit heart will get you through the day by working less.

Why we want more oxygen

When more oxygen is in our bodies, we burn fat, our breathing improves, our blood pressure goes down and our hearts work more efficiently. Oxygen also lowers triglycerides and cholesterol, increasing HDL, or "good" cholesterol, while decreasing LDL, or "bad" cholesterol. This means that your arteries will not be clogged and you may significantly decrease your risk of heart disease and stroke. More oxygen makes our brains work better, so we feel better. Studies show that depression is decreased when we increase oxygen flow into our bodies. Ancient techniques such as yoga, which specifically improve mental and spiritual well-being, achieve this by combining deep breathing and stretching, which improves oxygen and blood flow to specific parts of the body.

People who are active regularly have dramatically lower incidences of many cancers. Some research suggests that cancer cells thrive in an oxygen-depleted environment. The more oxygen in the bloodstream, the less hospitable you make your body to cancer. In addition, since many cancers are related to fat-soluble toxins, the less fat on your body, the less fat-soluble toxins your body can accumulate. The only kind of exercise that will burn fat is aerobic exercise because oxygen burns fat. The oxygen will burn your fat however you increase the oxygen flow in your body, through jumping around, increasing heart rate or employing an established deep-breathing technique.

The Western definition of aerobic

As mentioned above, an exercise is considered aerobic if it makes your heart beat faster than it normally does. When your heart is beating fast, you'll be breathing hard and sweating and will officially be in your "target zone" or "ideal range" (the kind of phrases that turn many people off). The point of working in the target range is to make your heart work harder than it usually does—that's how we strengthen any muscle.

There are official calculations you can do to find this target range. For example, it's said that by subtracting your age from 220, then multiplying that number by 60 percent, you will find your "threshold level"—which means "Your heart should be beating X beats per minute for 20 to 30 minutes." If you multiply the number by 75 percent, you will find your "ceiling level"—

which means "Your heart should not be beating faster than X beats per minute for 20 to 30 minutes." This is only an example. If you are on beta blockers (medications that slow your heart rate down), you'll want to make sure you discuss what target to aim for with your health professional.

Finding your pulse
You have pulse points all over your body. The easiest ones to find are those on your neck, at the base of your thumb, just below your earlobe or on your wrist. To check your heart rate, look at a watch or clock and begin to count your beats for 15 seconds (if the second hand is on the 12, count until it reaches 15). Then multiply by 4 to get your pulse.

Borg's Scale of Perceived Exertion (RPE)
This doesn't refer to the Borg on *Star Trek*, but to the Borg Scale of Perceived Exertion. This is a way of measuring exercise intensity without finding your pulse. Because of its simplicity, the RPE is now the recommended method for judging exertion.

The Borg scale measures activity from 6-20. Extremely light activity may rate a 7, for example, while a very, very strenuous activity may rate a 19. Exercise practitioners recommend that you do a "talk test" to rate your exertion, too. If you can't talk without gasping for air, you may be working too hard. You should be able to carry on a normal conversation throughout your activity. What's crucial to remember about RPE is that it is extremely individual; what one person judges to be a 7 someone else may judge to be a 10.

Other ways to increase oxygen flow
This will come as welcome news to people who have limited movement due to joint problems, arthritis or other conditions. You can increase the flow of oxygen into your bloodstream without exercising your heart muscle, by learning how to breathe deeply through your diaphragm. Many yoga-like programs and videos can teach you this technique, which does not require you to jump around. Deep breathing exercises will increase the oxygen flow into your bloodstream, which has many health benefits, including respiratory and stress reduction.

An aerobic activity versus active living
The phrase "aerobic activity" means that the *activity* causes your heart to pump harder and faster, and causes you to breathe faster, which increases oxygen flow. Activities such as cross-country skiing, walking, hiking and

biking are all aerobic. Exercise practitioners, however, hate the terms "aerobic activity" or "aerobics program" because it is not about what people do in their daily life. These terms have been replaced, to some degree, with the phrase "active living"—because that's what becoming unsedentary is all about.

There are many ways you can adopt an active lifestyle. Here are some suggestions:

- If you drive everywhere, pick the parking space farther away from your destination so you can work some daily walking into your life.
- If you take public transit everywhere, get off one or two stops early so you can walk the rest of the way to your destination.
- Take the stairs more often over escalators or elevators.
- Park at one side of the mall and then walk to the other.
- Take a stroll after dinner around your neighborhood.
- Volunteer to walk the dog.
- On weekends, go to the zoo or get out to flea markets, garage sales and so on.

Ways to become more active indoors include:

- Climbing stairs instead of taking elevators.
- Putting on music and dancing a little.
- Putting some small velcro weights around your ankles when you're doing chores.
- Using sacks of flour or sugar as "weights" to lift once or twice a day.
- Regularly cleaning out cupboards as an excuse to stretch and move.

LET'S GET PHYSICAL

Reports from the United States show that one out of three American adults are overweight, a sign of growing inactivity. Some people are so put off by the health club scene they become even more sedentary. Exercise failure is similar to diet failure, where you become so demoralized that you "cheat" and binge even more.

If you've been sedentary most of your life, there's nothing wrong with starting off with simple, even leisurely activities such as gardening, feeding the birds in a park or doing a few simple stretches. Any step you make toward being more active is a crucial and important one.

Experts also recommend that you find a friend, neighbor or relative to get physical with you. When your exercise plans include someone else, you'll be less apt to cancel plans or make excuses for not getting out there.

Things to Do Before "Moving Day"

When you decide to become more active, use this list as a gauge for pacing yourself. Start low and go slow.

1. Choose an activity that's right for you. Whether it's walking, chopping wood, jumping rope or folk dancing—pick something you enjoy. You don't have to do the same thing each time, either. Vary your routine to avoid monotony. Just make sure that whatever activity you choose is continuous for the duration. Walking for two minutes then stopping for three isn't continuous. It's also important to choose an activity that doesn't aggravate a pre-existing problem, such as eye problems. Lowering your head in a certain way (as in touching your toes), or straining your upper body can increase blood pressure and/or aggravate eye problems. If foot problems are a concern, perhaps an activity that doesn't involve walking, such as yoga, is better.

2. Choose the frequency. Decide how often you're going to do this activity. Twice, three, or four times a week? Or once a day? Try not to let two days pass without doing something. And pick a duration. If you're elderly or ill, even a few minutes is a good start. If you're sedentary but otherwise healthy, aim to build up to 20 to 30 minutes.

3. Choose the intensity level that's right for you. This is easy to do if you're using an exercise machine by just setting the dial. If you're walking, judge the intensity by how fast you are planning to walk, or how many hills you will be incorporating into your walk. In other words, how hard do you want your heart to beat?

4. Share your activity plans with your doctor. If you suffer from the following conditions, you may need to modify your plans:

    *   Diabetes
    *   Heart disease
    *   Osteoporosis
    *   High Blood Pressure

TEACHING CHILDREN ABOUT ACTIVE LIVING

You don't need to "teach" children to be active; they are born knowing how. We, in fact, teach them to become inactive through allowing them to engage in too many sedentary activities, such as watching television, sitting in front of the computer, or playing endless video games. We teach them inactivity by making them sit at a desk all day (which may not even be the best way to promote learning). We expose them to commercials that sell them sugar in the form of junk food and sugary soft drinks. Studies also show that physical activity is a clear deterrent from smoking and other substance abuse in the teenage population, and may also improve mental health, cutting down on mood disorders and teen suicides.

Obesity in childhood and adolescence is at an all-time high in North America. The American National Health and Nutrition Examination Survey III (NHANES III) revealed that 21 percent of people aged 12–19 were obese (i.e., their body weight exceeds the ideal weight for someone of their height by more than 20 percent), while as many as 40 percent of people in that age group were physically unfit. It wasn't until 1995 that the Dietary Guidelines for Americans even recommended physical activity. It's important to help your children establish an active lifestyle early—that will lower their risk for chronic illnesses and cancers.

How Local Governments Can Help

Urge your local levels of government to promote active living by expanding bicycle lanes and walking paths; creating car-free zones that enable pedestrians to walk freely; and preserving green space and conservation lands.

School-based activity programs
Those who grow up active tend to stay that way. Physical activity is a component of lifestyle, and lifestyle habits need to be established and reinforced throughout the school-age years if they are to be maintained later in life. When it comes to breast cancer, for example, evidence suggests that adverse factors early in life increase the risk, while the benefit of exercise in early life continues to work by reducing subsequent breast cancer risk. Make some of the following suggestions to your child's school:

- Make physical education mandatory throughout secondary school. In most school boards, just one credit in physical education is required at the secondary school level. This sends the message that physical education is not a priority, and is not valued in society. Making physical education a requirement at the secondary school level, in addition to nutrition or smoking education courses, may do wonders. You don't have to substitute gym credit for other credits; it should be made as mandatory as school attendance.
- Upgrade change rooms. The change room is often the reason so many

teens drop gym class. Private change stalls and showers can make a real difference for self-conscious teens, gay or lesbian teens, or teens concerned with under/overdeveloped bodies for their age and gender.

- De-emphasize competitive sports, and encourage "solitary" activities be given just as much value, such as walking, hiking or bicycling.

Physical activity means more outdoor activity, which is certainly a good thing. But because of ozone depletion, the great outdoors is not great without the right protection. Sun-safety education should be part of physical and health education for all children and teens. The sun is a major cause of skin cancers, which can be prevented with the right information at the right time of life. Chapter 5 provides more details about sun safety.

5
SUN SAFETY

By simply becoming educated about sun safety, we can prevent most skin cancers.

Skin cancer is a common type of neoplasm, or abnormal growth of tissue. There are two types of skin cancer: non-melanoma and melanoma. If recognized and treated, non-melanoma skin cancers are rarely fatal, though they can be disfiguring. And because they are often treated in the doctor's office, they are rarely registered (or tracked). Yet non-melanoma skin cancers are almost certainly the most common types of cancers for North Americans of both sexes.

A female friend of mine died from melanoma—the fatal skin cancer. It wasn't detected until it had spread to her brain. It is often missed and diagnosed too late because early stages of melanoma frequently have no symptoms. The incidence of melanoma is rising in both sexes, largely due to increased ultraviolet (UV) exposure. With the right information about sun safety in childhood, many melanomas can be prevented, too.

Did you know...

- The principal known cause of skin cancer is prolonged exposure to the sun's UV rays over several years, with most of the damage occurring during childhood.
- For most people, as much as 80 percent of their lifetime sun exposure has occurred by the time they are 20 years old.
- If children and teenagers protect themselves from the sun, they may significantly lessen their lifetime risk of developing skin cancer.

Source: Canadian Cancer Society, 2000

ANOTHER PREVENTABLE ENVIRONMENTAL CANCER

Skin cancer, like lung cancer, is an easily preventable environmental cancer. Unlike tobacco, however, the sun wasn't always as bad for you as it is today. It has become a serious health hazard due to all of the environmental pollutants that have damaged the ozone layer.

In the past, the ozone layer of the upper atmosphere protected the earth and its inhabitants from ultraviolet solar radiation. The ozone layer is made up of a band of ozone molecules that ultraviolet rays cannot usually penetrate. As synthetic chemicals (like chlorofluorocarbons) enter the stratosphere, however, solar radiation splits the ozone molecules into oxygen atoms. Some of these atoms then bond with the synthetic chemicals instead of regrouping, as they're supposed to, into ozone molecules once again. The result is a net loss of ozone and an increased penetration of ultraviolet radiation, something that just "wasn't supposed to happen."

Although the international community has responded to the crisis of ozone depletion by agreeing to phase out the production of most ozone-depleting substances, such as CFCs, the ozone layer will continue to thin for at least another 70 years. It is estimated that for every 1 percent decrease in ozone, we'll see a 3 percent rise in non-melanoma skin cancers.

Skin Cancers

Most forms of skin cancer are caused by repeated exposure to the sun's ultraviolet rays, which are categorized into A and B, known as UV-A and UV-B rays. The most damage is done during childhood. Evidence links non-melanoma skin cancer in particular to a combination of sun exposure, geographic location and genetic susceptibility. You're also at greater risk if you happen to be older, male, fair and freckled, with either blue or light-colored eyes.

The connection between sun exposure and malignant melanoma is not as clear-cut as the connection between sunlight and non-melanoma. While we do know that repeated sun exposure during childhood is a primary risk factor for malignant melanoma, establishing a direct link has so far proved impossible. As with non-melanoma skin cancers, your risk of melanoma increases if you have light hair, skin and eye color, and if you tend to burn easily. Your risk of melanoma increases even more if you have moles, freckles or red hair. In fact, the incidence of melanomas among fair-skinned populations is rising at a rate 3–6 percent higher than that of darker-skinned people. Moreover, higher rates of melanoma have been reported in geographic areas with lower latitudes, such as Australia.

Educating the Grown-Ups

We won't realize the fruits of sun-safety education for about 40 years, because most skin cancers are linked to early damaging exposure to sunlight. Before we can properly educate our children about sun safety, however, most of us need a refresher course, because a lot of us are misinformed.

Minimizing damaging exposure to the sun
The following are Sunsense Guidelines, published by the Canadian Cancer Society; these are considered universal sun-safety guidelines regardless of what country you live in!

1. Reduce sun exposure between 11 a.m. and 4 p.m. The sun's rays are the strongest between 11 a.m. and 4 p.m. If you can, plan your outdoor activities before or after this time. It's easy to remember this time—during these hours, your shadow is shorter than you are!

2. Seek shade or create your own shade. When you are outside, especially between 11 a.m. and 4 p.m., try to stay in the shade. Be prepared for places without any shade by taking along an umbrella. With an umbrella you can create shade wherever you need it.

3. Slip! On clothing to cover your arms and legs. Covering your skin will protect it from the sun. Choose clothing that is loose fitting, tightly woven, lightweight.

4. Slap! On a wide-brimmed hat. Most skin cancers occur on the face and neck, so this area needs extra protection. Wear a hat with a wide brim that covers your head, face, ears and neck. Hats without a wide brim, like baseball caps, do not give you enough protection.

5. Slop! On a sunscreen with a Sun Protection Factor (SPF) of #15 or higher. Look for "broad spectrum" on the label. This means that the sunscreen offers protection against two types of ultraviolet rays, UV-A and UV-B. Apply sunscreen generously 20 minutes before outdoor activities. Reapply frequently, at least every two hours, and after swimming or exercise that makes you perspire. No sunscreen can absorb all of the sun's rays. Use sunscreen along with shade, clothing and hats, not instead of them. Use sunscreen as a back-up in your sun protection plan.

6. Keep babies under one year out of the direct sun. Babies need extra protection because their skin is very sensitive. Keep your child's stroller,

playpen or carriage in the shade.

7. Tanning parlors and sunlamps are not a safe way to tan. Tanning salons do not give you a "safe tan without burning." No tan is a safe tan. A tan is evidence of sun damage. Just like the sun, tanning lights and sun lamps emit ultraviolet rays that can cause sunburn and aging skin, and increase your risk of skin cancer. The strength of the ultraviolet rays, especially the UV-A type, may actually be higher in tanning beds than in sunlight!

8. Wear sunglasses. Sunglasses can help prevent damage to your eyes by blocking a large amount of ultraviolet rays. Keep your "shades" on, and make sure your children wear them, too! Choose sunglasses with even shading, medium to dark lenses (grey, brown or green tint), UV-A and UV-B protection. These qualities can be found in many inexpensive sunglasses.

9. Check your skin regularly. Most skin cancers can be cured, if caught early enough. Get to know your skin! Know the location and appearance of birthmarks and moles. Check your skin regularly so you can detect any changes. See your doctor right away if you notice:

    •   a birthmark or mole that changes shape, colour, size or surface
    •   a sore that does not heal
    •   new growths on your skin
    •   patches of skin that bleed, ooze, swell, itch or become red or bumpy.

Add to this list medication checks. Check all your medications to see if they can make you oversensitive to sunlight, a common but once considered minor side effect. Did you know, for example, that even the popular nerve herb St. John's wort makes you more sensitive to sunlight? Antibiotics are also classic culprits. Did you know, too, that sunscreens are misused? They are not designed for sun-worshipping, but for minimizing exposure to the sun when you're out doing normal activities.

We need more public education to encourage North Americans to adopt sun-safety guidelines. We also need to make sure that parents and caregivers are getting the right sun-safety messages.

How consumer power can help
Consumers have a lot of power. Here are some ways we can exercise it:

1. Get some other concerned parents together and lobby your school board to do sun-safety education as part of its health education initia-

tives (right along with anti-smoking, physical activity and nutrition education).

2. In addition, encourage your child's school to practice sun safety by adopting the following policies:

- When the ultraviolet (UV) index is high, schools should plan indoor alternatives to outdoor activities.
- Grassy areas should replace paved schoolyards. The classic grade school play area is paved with concrete or asphalt, which reflect harmful UV rays. Grass is preferred; trees should be added for shade.

3. Contact your local government and request that more shaded areas be created at beaches and other outdoor public places frequented by children and young adults.

4. Contact the manufacturers of your favorite brand of sunscreen and suggest they use some of their public relations dollars on sun-safety campaigns that target parents or caregivers of young children. Remind them that by informing the public about how important their product is, they'll sell more product!

5. Contact other sun product manufacturers (sunglasses, sun hats or visors) who stand to sell more product by selling protection, too.

6. Contact children's clothing companies and request that they design and manufacture sun-protective clothing.

7. Contact the manufacturers of drugs that cause oversensitivity to the sun, and request that they always include the information in their advertising.

Occupational sunlight
Anyone who works outdoors is being exposed to an environmental hazard: the sun. Public-utility workers in Maryland, for example, whose work involves extensive exposure to sunlight, were found to be at greater risk of squamous cell carcinoma, a common type of skin cancer, and actinic keratosis, another common type of skin cancer. A British study also confirmed the cancer risks associated with prolonged occupational exposure to sunlight. In addition to an increased incidence of squamous cell carcinoma and basal cell carcinoma, British outdoor workers experienced all sorts of melanomas of skin that had been exposed, such as on the head, face and neck.

To minimize the impact of prolonged sun exposure among outdoor workers, companies employing outdoor workers should join forces with their state departments or provincial ministries of labor to provide sun-safety gear to all outdoor workers (sunscreen and hats, and protective clothing, such as long-sleeved cotton shirts); shaded areas on-site for breaks; sun-safety education about appropriate use of sunscreen, and how to do spot checks (checking for unusual changes on the skin, which often appear as spots or moles).

Protective Clothing

Canadian designer Linda Lundstrum was one of the first fashion designers to make sun-safety clothing. Although her line targets wealthier women who want to vacation in the sun, she's on the right track. There is a real demand for lightweight fabric clothing that can block harmful UV-B rays. Most of us have the wardrobe already, which consists of a wide-brimmed hat; cotton pants, longer skirts or dresses; and clothing made of a denser weave of fabric, such as cotton.

Many of us, however, find these clothes too hot for very warm summer days. So what's needed are manufacturers of clothing using an ultraprotective, lightweight fabric offering UV protection in designs that will make us want to wear protective clothing. Contact some local designers, retailers or schools of fashion design and suggest that sun-safety lines be designed and competitively priced so that consumers can afford these clothes.

Departments or ministries of health can get involved by instituting labeling that designates certain clothing "sun-safe," so we know what we're buying.

SUNSCREENS AND SMOKE SCREENS

Most of us don't understand how to use sunscreen properly, or even what the purpose of a sunscreen is. Sunscreens are classified according to how well they prevent sunburn. The higher the number, the greater the protection. They may also prevent sun-induced pigmentation changes, such as tanning, freckling, and sun spots; photodamage at the DNA level; or wrinkling and skin cancer.

Sunscreens have been shown to reduce rates of actinic keratoses, a type of skin cancer in humans. In theory, this could mean a reduction in rates of squamous cell carcinoma as well. Some have estimated that if sunscreen is used regularly in the first 18 years of life, the lifetime risk of non-melanoma skin cancer would be reduced by an impressive 78 percent.

The problem with commercial sunscreens is that they encourage a false sense of security. Sun worshippers continue to spend hours on the beach, confident that their sunscreens have made them safe. In reality, there are other, more effective countermeasures against skin damage (like wearing protective clothing and sitting in the shade), but we haven't seen these measures marketed with the vengeance of sunscreen.

Sunscreen Safety Campaigns

Sunscreen manufacturers ought to include information about what their product does and what it does not do in their advertising. Sunscreens are certainly one measure we can use to reduce skin cancers, but they are not the only measure, and the public needs to be made aware of this fact. Sunscreen advertising campaigns should also include instructions on sunscreen application and usage; at the moment, this information languishes in tiny print on the packaging. Many people forget to reapply sunscreen after swimming, sweating or showering. Many people do not know how to efficiently apply sunscreen so that the whole body is protected. There is room for sunscreen "aid" products—products that help you get to hard-to-reach places on the back—that can help to evenly apply it.

Local governments can help by making sunscreen readily available and affordable to low-income people at local parks and recreation sites. For example, in Australia, sunscreen is handed out at public beaches and outdoor recreational facilities as part of ongoing public education campaigns aimed at reducing that country's high rate of skin cancer. Since people will still be out in the sun (we're human, and we seek sunlight), widespread use of sunscreen ought to be available to everyone.

SUN AND DAUGHTERS

Caucasian women are particularly vulnerable to sun damage because of deeply entrenched messages from the media and our culture about beauty, body image and the attractiveness of a suntan. (This is in contrast, however, to conflicting messages about beauty for women of colour, who are told that lighter skin is more attractive.) In a recent British documentary, women admitted that they felt more attractive and thinner with a tan. The motivations for tanning are not unlike motivations for smoking, rooted in body image and beauty standards (see chapters 2 and 3). However, there are safer techniques for achieving a tan that do not involve direct exposure to sunlight. Although it would be safer to change the messages women receive about suntans and beauty, in the meantime, we need to encourage our daughters to at least look for safe tanning methods. Check with your dermatologist or family doctor about the safety of self-tanning lotions as an alternative to tanning beds and salons, which cancer experts declare unsafe.

Hazards of Sunlight Deprivation

We need some sunlight; and women, in particular, need some sunlight for bone health, as vitamin D is activated in their bodies by a little sunlight, and women are more at risk than men for osteoporosis. Fifteen minutes of natural sunlight a day is all women need, and if their skin is exposed, wearing sunscreen for these intervals is fine. In fact, lack of sunlight can result in both sexes (but more commonly in women) in Seasonal Affective Disorder (SAD), a form of depression or low mood that results from being light-deprived.

VACATIONS IN THE SUN

To get the sun-safety message out to the public, consumers should urge the vacation and travel industries to join forces. Tour companies selling sun vacation travel should be encouraged to spend some of their advertising and promotion budget on sun-safety education. Websites or travel agencies could offer sun-safety pamphlets for travellers. "Sun Safety in the Caribbean" brochures, for example, could be jointly funded by travel bureaus, airlines, package tour operators and departments/ ministries of tourism. Such brochures could include official guidelines for sun safety, as well as reminders for travelers to check their medications for sun-sensitivity side effects.

If you're planning to vacation in the sun, bring along plenty of sunscreen with proper instructions for use, and plan alternative activities for peak sun hours. As a consumer, encourage the travel and tourism industry to help you protect yourself. You know the drill by now: email, fax or write the appropriate travel agent you deal with and make your preferences known.

It's disturbing to think of something so natural and beautiful as sun as a hazard. Chapters 7, 8 and 9 will help to explain this by discussing the destructive chemicals that are ruining the environment and our health. In this chapter we learned that some people are more vulnerable to the hazards of excessive sun exposure than others because they work outdoors. The carcinogenic soup to which many of us are unwittingly exposed in our workplaces also contributes to a variety of cancers, and may be the trigger that trips our cancer switches. If that's the case, what is the role of genes in cancer? The answer, provided in the next chapter, may surprise you.

6
OUR GENES

What is the role of our genes in stopping cancer at the source? Scientists have reported finding genes for various diseases, which has led people to believe that having a particular gene means that they will get a particular disease. This is not true. You can stop the top killer chronic diseases (heart disease, stroke and Type 2 diabetes) and the top killer cancers (lung cancer and colon cancer) at the source by modifying your lifestyle—changing your dietary habits and levels of activity. In other words, what your genes are exposed to has more impact on your cancer risk than simply having the genes.

If you smoke (see chapter 2), consume a diet that is low in nutrients and high in fat (see chapter 3), drink alcohol to the point of liver damage (see chapter 3), are completely inactive (see chapter 4), or spend hours in the sun without protecting yourself (see chapter 5), your cancer risk may increase whether you have certain cancer genes or not. At birth, our genes are like a bunch of light switches in the Off position. Certain triggers, such as food, tobacco or other toxins (see chapters 7, 8 and 9) can turn these switches to the On position. If you have a "lung cancer gene," so what? If you don't smoke, you won't turn on that switch. The genetic link is often meaningless when we're looking at stopping cancers at the source.

This chapter takes a closer look at what having certain genes means. It also explores the controversial issues involved with genetic testing, something that more and more people may be interested in now that the Human Genome Project, an international project whereby scientists have mapped all of our genes, is complete.

THE ROLE OF GENES IN CANCER

Stopping Cancer at the Source

We are now quite certain that most cancers occur because of a change in the genetic makeup of cells when they become cancerous. The genes involved in cancer are normal genes that have both tumor-inducing and tumor-suppressing functions. In other words, these are normal genes that can be altered by cancer-causing substances or agents we call *carcinogens*, such as tobacco.

Most experts believe cancers are triggered by an interaction between lifestyle habits and genes (smoking, drinking, eating, exercise and sun-exposure habits), and planetary habits and genes (meaning the air and water around us that we cannot control). When it comes to stopping cancer at the source, the challenge continues to be about recognizing what in our personal lives and the environment we inhabit needs to be modified, avoided or eliminated to ensure that genetic damage and resulting cancers do not occur.

What it Means to Carry a Cancer Gene

When you're told you carry a gene for a particular cancer it means that you have inherited a normal gene that is more vulnerable to "attack" by certain carcinogens, meaning that it can mutate. Cancers that are considered to be familial (inherited) are cancers that occur in first-degree relatives (parents, siblings and children). Grandmothers, great-aunts and paternal relatives are not as crucial in determining familial cancers. Genetic screening can find some of these vulnerable genes, but what does this information mean?

Having the colon cancer gene
There is a colon cancer gene, but the presence of a genetic mutation for colon cancer does not mean you will get colon cancer, nor does the absence of a genetic mutation mean that you will *not* get colon cancer. Therefore, genetic screening for colon cancer is not meaningful information for most people. And the stress a positive test can generate may cause more harm than good.

Most colon cancer comes from a polyp, a small benign growth that can sprout into colon cancer, but when found early, can be removed. There is one type of colon cancer, however, that does not originate from polyps, known as hereditary non-polyposis colorectal cancer (HNPCC). This is a hereditary colon cancer that strikes at about age 45. People with the gene that causes this cancer may also be at greater risk for cancer of the uterus, bladder or ureter (the orifice out of which we urinate), pancreas and stomach. Roughly 5 percent of colorectal cancer is due to an HNPCC gene mutation.

A second gene mutation has been discovered in approximately 6 percent of the Ashkenazi Jewish population (Jews of Eastern European descent). If you are not Jewish, it is exceedingly rare to test positive for this second kind of mutation. Finally, less than 1 percent of colon cancer, known as familial adenomatous polyposis (FAP), which is characterized by hundreds of polyps, is linked to a rare genetic mutation.

So, what can you do if you test positive for one of these genes? Not much more than anyone else in the population, whose risk of colon cancer after 45 is significant due simply to age and lifestyle habits. All you can do if you test positive for a genetic mutation for colon cancer is to be screened more frequently than people who do not have a genetic mutation for colon cancer. Stopping colon cancer at the source can be done through modifying your personal habits.

Having the breast cancer gene
Familial breast cancer accounts for only about 5 percent of all breast cancers overall, but in younger women it is implicated in 25 percent of cases. Several inherited genes can cause susceptibility to this cancer, including BRCA1, BRCA2, BRCA3, hMlH1 and hMLH2. The most well-known breast cancer gene that has been isolated is BRCA1. Women who have this gene are more susceptible to breast cancer than those who don't.

It is possible to be screened for BRCA1, but doing mass screenings is not very useful because this gene accounts for only 4–5 percent of all breast cancers. It is also found in women who don't get breast cancer and in women who come from low-risk families. And since we don't know what finding BRCA1 in a woman without a high-risk family means, screening everyone could wind up scaring people for no good reason. Another problem with screening is that there is no way to tell a woman who doesn't test positive for the BRCA1 gene that she's not at risk for breast cancer since there are so many other factors involved, such as diet, activity level and exposure to environmental toxins.

If you are BRCA1-positive, it's estimated, using data from high-risk families, that there is an 85 percent chance of your developing breast cancer before age 80, although about 50 percent of women who fall into this group will develop the disease before they are 50. It has also been found that women who are BRCA1-positive come from families in which 50 percent of all female members are affected. If you have BRCA1 and come from a low-risk family, nobody knows for sure what this means, if indeed it means anything at all.

There are some extreme prevention therapies now recommended to women who test positive for this gene, including having a prophylactic bilateral mastectomy (removing both healthy breasts), taking powerful anti-estrogen drugs, which can cause dramatic side effects, or doing the same thing all women do—regular breast exams in your doctor's office, breast self-examination (BSE) and mammography at regular intervals.

SHOULD YOU GO FOR GENETIC TESTING?

The problem with finding out whether you have a mutated gene that could cause cancer in your body is that it is not necessarily meaningful information. The stress that the information causes could be more damaging to you than the mutated gene. On the other hand, knowing you are vulnerable to certain cancers may motivate you to modify your lifestyle—to change your diet or incorporate more activity into your daily routine.

A wider issue surrounding genetic testing is the fast-approaching future: a future where a long list of genetic information may be compiled about each person. And that means there may be a stigma attached to certain information getting out to people who may not understand what having a certain gene means, and who may discriminate against you for having certain cancer genes. This is not an issue that you need to worry about today, but it may be one that will affect your children ten years from now. Now that the Human Genome Project is complete, many more cancer gene tests will be available.

The Downside of Genetic Testing

Testing for genetic mutations will produce a database of confidential information that can be abused. Here are some questions medical ethicists are asking today:

1. Who owns this information? It is currently unclear whether this information is for you and your doctor's eyes only. Would you want other family members to find out about your genes? How about your employer?

2. How will this information be used? The film Gattaca dramatizes the results of a genetically obsessed culture. In this film, one's genetic makeup determines eligibility for education, employment and social status, even though the film's protagonist makes it clear that "genoism" (a word that in the film means discrimination against people with

genetic defects or mutations) is against the law. Gattaca shows us a world where every strand of hair or eyelash serves as one's genetic resumé.

Insurance companies in the United States already practice a form of genoism with clauses that prevent people with "pre-existing conditions" from receiving health care insurance. Does this mean health insurers in the near future could require, for example, BRCA-positive women to undergo breast removal surgery as a condition of coverage? Or would health insurance premiums simply become unaffordable for BRCA-positive women, or the families of these women? Or would employers demand this surgery prior to hiring?

3. Designer babies. How does knowing about certain cancer genes affect our motivation to "design" our babies? Would cancer gene testing become available prenatally? Are fetuses with certain cancer genes likely to be aborted for these reasons? In India, for example, female fetuses are often aborted because they are viewed as economic burdens on families; similarly, little girls who grow up to be breast cancer patients may be viewed as economic burdens.

4. Do we understand our test results? Critics of genetic testing state that misunderstood genetic information can do enormous damage. What happens if we have inadequate genetic counseling? It's important to consider the following before deciding to get tested:

- Testing Negative. Testing negative is never a "true negative" since the test is not an accurate prediction of one's future health. Some mistakenly interpret a negative result to mean that they will never develop cancer. If several family members are being tested at once, those in the family who test negative may suffer from "survivor's guilt" if others test positive.

- Testing Positive. On the flip side, testing positive is not necessarily a guarantee of developing cancer. Healthy people who are told they have a "ticking bomb" gene could needlessly suffer from anxiety, depression, hopelessness and strained relationships with family members.

- Rich versus Poor. Already, genetic tests are not always covered by the government, and in the future, they may be considered "extra." This may mean that some people will have access to genetic information because of their income levels, while others will have no access to it. Currently prenatal testing is already unevenly distributed; more affluent communities have more access to testing than poor communities.

The Upside of Genetic Testing

As mentioned above, if you know you have the potential for certain cancers, you may be much more likely to modify your personal habits to help stop certain cancers at the source, such as lung, colon or skin cancers. And, if you know you have the potential for certain estrogen-dependent cancers, you may also help to stop those cancers at the source by consuming a diet that keeps you lean and healthy.

Knowing how various carcinogens can attack genes and cause them to mutate can also influence our decisions about some of the wider toxins we're exposed to—toxins we cannot control—such as those found in air and water. If we are aware of the triggers that may switch on a cancer gene, we may decide that working at a nuclear power plant is not such a good idea. Or we may decide not to buy a house that sits on top of a hazardous-waste site. Fully informed about environmental toxins, we may be more apt to help get rid of toxins in the global fight to stop cancer at the source.

PART II

WHAT'S POLITICAL

Stopping Cancer at the Source

No one in industry or government woke up one morning and said: "Let's make money and ruin the earth." In other words, you and I bear some responsibility in this mess we've made of our planet. One of the reasons it's so difficult to get rid of many cancer-causing environmental pollutants is that we, as consumers, depend on so many products that necessitate their production and emissions. I refer to this as our collective "chemical dependency." The manufacturing of plastic, for example, used in an infinite variety of products, releases carcinogenic chemicals. We need alternatives to the products we've come to rely on, and manufacturers need incentives to create those alternatives.

For the sake of our environment, we've had to part with some products we loved. Aerosol sprays, for example, have been removed from the marketplace. We've also largely done away with the production of ozone-destroying chlorofluorocarbons (CFCs), used in refrigeration, air-conditioning systems, and dozens of other products. At first, both consumers and industry contended that CFCs were irreplaceable, and that stopping their manufacture would deprive us of our standard of living. We screamed: "There are no available substitutes;" "It will cost us thousands of jobs." But as the ozone depletion problem persisted, public concern helped to eliminate CFCs. By the mid-1990s, levels of CFCs were significantly reduced in the upper atmosphere, and industry accelerated the phasing out of CFCs in their products. By the year 2015, CFCs will be virtually eliminated, a goal which once seemed impossible. And lo and behold, substitutes for CFCs were developed and replacement products are being made with those substitute processes.

The bottom line is that when given the incentives, manufacturers can be very creative in finding solutions and, in the process, can open new markets and opportunities as well. Indeed, if we can invent ingenious ways to destroy the earth, we can re-invent ways to reverse that destruction. If we let our voices be heard by government and industry, we can help solve problems of environmental degradation.

Chapters 7, 8 and 9 discuss the carcinogenic agents that are in our environment—workplace, air, water, soil, food chain—and beyond our personal control.

7
THE HAZARDS OF WORKING FOR A LIVING

O ccupational hazards were the topic of the much-publicized film, *Erin Brokovich*, starring Julia Roberts. This film has helped to bring attention to cancers and diseases caused by industrial carcinogens.

One of the most infamous examples of workplace-related cancers can be seen in the "Bell Cluster." Between April 1995 and September 1996, eight Bell Canada employees in their thirties, who were hired within similar time frames, and who worked close to one another on the same floor, were diagnosed with cancer: five with breast cancer, two with colon cancer and one with brain cancer. None of these cancer patients had strong or remarkable family histories of their cancers. The incidence was more than 12 times what would be considered normal in this 30-something age group.

This bizarre phenomenon, which seemed to be more than coincidental, became known as the Bell Cluster. These employees (some have since passed away) insist that their cancers are linked to emissions from their computer equipment, which they say were magnified due to the crowded conditions in which they were working. But since research on the relationship between cancer and electromagnetic fields is inconclusive, there is no way to prove the link.

Claims filed by the Bell Cluster employees were rejected by the then–Workers' Compensation Board (now known in Ontario as the Workplace Safety and Insurance Board); an epidemiologist hired by Bell Canada concluded that the Bell Cluster was "random"—meaning that the cancer diagnoses were coincidental and not linked to any one thing. Survivors of the Bell Cluster want Canada to insist on stringent standards for computer equipment and other sources of electromagnetic radiation, believing it best to err on the side of caution. The Bell Cluster story, infamous in Canadian occupational health circles, tells us more about what we don't know and can't prove, but strongly suspect. It illustrates the frustration that cancer prevention advocates face when trying to get industry to take action to protect workers.

You're more likely to be affected by workplace carcinogens if you work or live in energy-sealed buildings; are exposed to fumes from carpets, pesticides, cleaners and airborne allergens; are exposed to industrial chemicals, such as those found in plants that process wood, metal, plastics, paints and textiles; are in constant contact with pesticides, fungicides and fertilizers; live in high-pollution areas; and work in dry cleaning, hair salons, pest control, printing and photocopying.

This chapter is not about what we don't know and can't prove; it is limited to what we do know and can prove about occupational hazards as of this writing. One of the problems is that there is a dearth of conclusive scientific evidence to prove cause and effect in the area of occupational carcinogens. It's also important to note that this chapter informs you about carcinogens in the workplace; it does not cover suspected or known carcinogens in the home, a vast topic that warrants a separate book, although it does discuss workplace-home crossovers. For specific information about indoor toxins, such as radon gas, see the resource list at the back of this book.

WHAT WE DO KNOW—AND CAN PROVE

In the past, occupational exposure to carcinogens was often severe, and involved very direct exposure to carcinogens. In the 1880s, coal miners would inevitably die of lung cancer (known as black lung disease) before the hazard was recognized and controlled through changes in the mining industry and the introduction of protective gear. In areas where we could prove a link between a substance in the workplace and cancer, we got better at removing hazards or protecting workers from those hazards.

For many working North Americans, retirement won't involve more golfing or home decorating; it will involve trips to the hospital for cancer treatment. Occupationally induced cancers will continue to afflict those who entered the workforce before proper controls were introduced. As consumers, we are all affected by industrial hazards since so many of the chemicals in high use have never been tested for human health safety. An arsenal of new chemicals is introduced each year, which puts all of us at risk. In fact, many of the existing chemicals in high use haven't been tested either.

In a 1999 report on occupational hazards, it was noted that occupational cancers are not evenly distributed throughout the population. Blue-collar workers such as those in agriculture, mining, metal working and painting have five times the rate of occupational cancers. In 1995, Dr. Peter Inante, Director of the Office of Standards Review, Occupational Safety and Health Administration of the U.S. Department of Labor, stated that blue-collar workers "appeared to be the canaries in our society for identifying human chemical carcinogens in the general environment." It's crucial to note, too, that non-unionized workers in Canada and the United States have less access to information on occupational hazards and are also at greater risk.

Here is what we know so far regarding workplace carcinogens, discussed in alphabetical order:

Agriculture-Related Carcinogens

Concern is growing about the dangers of repeated exposure to herbicides and pesticides. Because of the way food is grown and processed in the West, these chemicals are familiar to just about everyone who shops at their local supermarket. They are of special relevance to people who work in the agricultural industry: greenhouse workers, veterinarians, pesticide applicators, pesticide manufacturers and anyone around pesticides in non-occupational settings are exposed to these chemicals.

The risk of lymphoma, where cancer spreads through the lymph nodes, for example, has increased among agricultural workers. And in Canada, a study of Saskatchewan farmers found a significant association between risk of non-Hodgkin's lymphoma and farmland sprayed with herbicides. One umbrella examination of 20 different studies spanning eight countries found that, compared to the general population, farmers suffer from higher rates of Hodgkin's disease, multiple myeloma, leukemia, skin cancers and cancers of the lip, stomach and prostate. A 1999 Swedish study found that the 400 patients involved with non-Hodgkins lymphoma were 60 percent more likely to report exposures to herbicides and three times more likely to report exposures to fungicides. Note: exposure to pesticides and herbicides in home gardening results in the same risks.

Asbestos

Asbestos is a naturally occurring mineral that was used to manufacture products such as cement, fireproof textiles, paper, brake linings, vinyl floor tiles, additives for asphalt, resins, plastics and sealants. It was also used widely for building insulation. The Johns-Manville plant in Scarborough, Ontario, which manufactured asbestos-cement pipe from 1948 to 1980, was labeled a "world-class occupational health disaster" by the Royal Commission on Matters of Health Arising from the Use of Asbestos in Ontario back in 1984. In Sarnia, Ontario, home of the Holmes Caposite plant, asbestos levels were the highest ever encountered. Even as early as 1958, this employer and the government were aware of the health risks associated with asbestos. A 1987 study found a sixfold increase in lung cancer amongst Holmes workers, while families of Holmes workers are being diagnosed with mesothelioma, an asbestos-related lung cancer.

Anyone working in old buildings with asbestos is at greater risk for a variety of cancers, including lung and gastrointestinal cancers. Severe asbestos exposure, for example, can double the risk of stomach and colorectal cancer, although the cancer can take more than 20 years to develop. Unfortunately, because of the time lapse between exposure and development of the disease, it is hard to link these cancers to asbestos exposure in any conclusive way, although experts maintain that asbestos can be the cause. Note: exposure to asbestos in the home results in the same risks.

Dioxin

Dioxin is considered a known human carcinogen and is associated with higher rates of all kinds of cancers. This substance is an environmental estrogen (see chapter 8) associated with higher rates of reproductive cancers, and is a by-product of any chlorinated compound. In other words, dioxins are not produced intentionally; when chlorinated compounds break down, dioxin is the result. Dioxin, therefore, is a waste product. Those who work in the plastics industry, or are exposed to bleached paper or incinerators, are exposed to dioxin.

Environmental Tobacco Smoke (ETS)

As we saw in chapter 2, anyone who works in an environment where s/he is exposed to second-hand smoke is at greater risk for lung cancer and possibly other cancers, such as breast cancer. Some occupational exposures are exacerbated by cigarette smoke, especially asbestos and radon. This complicates matters because it's hard enough to isolate certain carcinogens, but when they attack us in combination, we don't have the scientific measurement techniques in place to track multiple factors appropriately. Note:

exposure to ETS in the home results in the same risks.

Metalworking Fluids

Metalworking fluids are the mineral oils, cutting oils, lubricating oils and coolants used in industries that perform machining, grinding or forming processes. These substances are linked to an increased risk of cancer of the larynx, rectum, pancreas, skin, scrotum and bladder. Untreated or mildly treated mineral oils are known carcinogens. Vegetable-based oils are an alternative lubricant to mineral oils and a number of workplaces are using this substitute.

Methylene Chloride

Methylene chloride is a liquid used in food, furniture and plastics processing, as well as in paint removing. This substance is labeled as a probable human carcinogen by the U.S. Environmental Protection Agency (EPA) and has been determined to be toxic under the Canadian Environmental Protection Act. Methylene chloride can also cross the placenta and affect fetal development. In 1997, according to the National Pollutants Release Inventory, there were still more than 23,000 kilograms of methylene chloride released in Toronto alone. Comparable levels of methylene chloride are no doubt in all major urban centers across the United States.

Mining Industry–Related Carcinogens

Sudbury, Ontario, the mining capital of Canada, has seen countless well-documented examples of occupational exposure to lung carcinogens like asbestos and radiation in mines. The process involved in nickel refining is also dangerous, though foundry workers, gold miners and those exposed to chromate are probably at equal risk. For some hard-rock miners the risk is more pronounced, particularly for nickel and gold miners who were in the workforce prior to 1945. And while it is suspected that the risk in hard-rock miners may in part be due to exposure to radon, there is some evidence that silica may be a carcinogen in its own right. Arsenic, among other culprits, may also have been present.

Perchloroethylene

Known as "perc," this is the infamous carcinogen associated with dry-cleaning establishments. Perc is used in its vapor or gas form to clean clothes, and has been identified as a probable carcinogen associated with higher rates of cancers of all kinds. Workers in dry-cleaning establishments are at

greatest risk, but since so many dry cleaners are located in residential neighborhoods or in multi-use buildings such as apartment complexes, we are all
exposed to perc when the vapors are not properly contained. Almost all
perc vapors escape into the air. Even when you pick up dry-cleaned clothes,
you're exposed to low levels of perc.

Perc is also used as a metal degreaser and an ingredient in many chemicals. To date, governments have failed to act on recommendations to find
alternative cleaning processes to dry cleaning.

Petroleum Industry–Related Carcinogens

There are a number of risks associated with the use or manufacture of
petroleum. The following carcinogens are associated with petroleum and
other industries:

Benzene
Occupational exposure to benzene, which is a component of gasoline and
of some new building adhesives, is thought to cause leukemia. When lead
was banned from gasoline, additional benzene was put in some gasoline as
an additive. It is also used as a solvent for other petrochemicals such as
paint, certain plastics, foams and pesticides.

Workers in the oil and chemical industries are at risk, as well as fire-
fighters, who face benzene exposure as a contaminant in fire smoke.
Consumers are exposed to benzene through tailpipe emissions from cars,
and engines found on lawnmowers or leaf-blowers, as well as evaporated
gasoline. There are currently no air quality standards in place for benzene.

Diesel exhaust
Diesel exhaust is considered a probable human carcinogen, and is associated with higher rates of lung cancers in occupational groups exposed to
diesel exhaust. Diesel is used in some workplaces to provide electrical
power from generators, but the major source of occupational exposure is to
public transit workers, taxi and truck drivers and workers in shipping and
handling areas where diesel vehicles idle.

Polycyclic Aromatic Hydrocarbons (PAHs)
PAHs are chemicals that are released whenever fuels such as oil, gasoline,
coal and wood are burned. Most of us are exposed to PAHs through emissions from cars, coal-fired generating stations, municipal incinerators,
home heating and industrial furnaces. Workers in foundries, in aluminum
or coke production, in petroleum refining, and workers exposed to asphalt

have higher risks of cancer of the esophagus, pancreas, prostate and lung. It's hard to isolate PAHs as a single carcinogen because they're always mixed with other substances. PAHs are one of the most potent environmental pollutants.

Radiation

Radiation is a risk factor for leukemia. We don't yet know how this risk will affect nuclear energy workers. However, those same workers have displayed some signs of exposure to electromagnetic fields (EMF), and that kind of

---

Known carcinogens at the office (or home) may be found in:

- Asbestos building materials
- Cleaning products and disinfectants
- Urea-formaldehyde foam insulation
- Adhesives (may contain naphthalene, phenol, ethanol, vinyl chloride, formaldehyde, acrylonitrile and epoxy, which are toxic substances that release vapors)
- Toners used in copy machines and printers
- Particleboard furniture and space dividers
- Permanent-ink pens and markers (contain acetone, cresol, ethnol, phenol, toluene and xylene)
- Polystyrene cups
- Second-hand smoke
- Synthetic office carpet (may contain acrylic, polyester and nylon plastic fibers, and formaldehyde-based finishes, pesticides due to moth-proofing for wool only)
- Correction fluid (may contain cresol, ethanol, trichloroethlyene and naphthalene, which are all toxic chemicals)

---

exposure is thought to be another cause of leukemia. There is a reputed link between brain tumors and proximity to electromagnetic fields, but this connection is still being investigated. Lymphoma is another one of the malignancies that has been linked to exposure to electromagnetic fields, but nuclear energy workers did not show significant association with lymphoma in studies done to date. Nor is there conclusive proof of EMF causing the Bell Cluster cancers, discussed at the beginning of this chapter.

HOW DO WE PROTECT OURSELVES FROM WORKPLACE CARCINOGENS?

Since so many environmental carcinogens originate in the workplace, and are then emitted into the air, water or land, eliminating carcinogens in the

For More Information...

Specific concerns can be explored through the NIOSH-TIC database, maintained by the U.S. National Institute of Occupational Safety and Health (NIOSH), available at various university and public libraries. NIOSH Information Dissemination can also be accessed directly by calling 513-533-8287. Finally, the Centers for Disease Control (CDC) in Atlanta, Georgia, (404-639-3311) can be consulted. In Canada, the Toxicological Index database (Infotox) provides peer-reviewed information concerning chemicals identified in the workplace.

workplace—at the source—would have a huge impact on cleaning up the environment in general.

A woefully inadequate body of knowledge exists about workplace carcinogens. In urban centers, residents are exposed to a wide array of carcinogens in their workplaces, but there is only clear evidence of the cancer-causing potential for nine substances (known as the Noxious Nine): benzene, diesel exhaust, polycyclic aromatic hydrocarbons, perchloroethylene, dioxin, pesticides, metalworking fluids, methylene chloride and asbestos. As for the rest of the long list of suspected carcinogens, researchers point to the need for "more research in the future." The most important investigation into workplace carcinogens is the ongoing review process at the International Agency for Research on Cancer. This material is reproduced at the end of chapter 8.

The absence of information or conclusive proof is not the same thing as the absence of risk. Many cancer experts assert that the goal of industry ought to be zero risk in the workplace by taking a precautionary or "seat belt" approach. For instance, wearing a seat belt in a car is a precautionary approach; we don't know for sure we'll have an accident, but we have enough evidence to know that we must be careful on the roads. Similarly, we can prevent the risk of carcinogen exposure by not allowing untested substances to be used until proven safe.

You'd think that by now we could simply ban known workplace carcinogens and use our scientific knowledge to find substitutes. Sometimes the only way to do this is to ban the worker instead of the substance. If a carcinogenic substance is essential to the manufacturing process, protective clothing and other equipment, as well as improved ventilation systems (such as those used in the mining industry) are ways to control exposure.

Thus, carcinogenic exposure in the workplace has been reduced to the extent where it can no longer be proven that workers are at any greater risk than the general public. This is the case, for example, with hard-rock miners. It does seem plausible, in such circumstances, that those who joined the workforce in the last few years are at no greater risk of occupationally induced cancers than the rest of us.

Government's Response

What protections are in place for workers when it comes to workplace carcinogens?

Compensation
Governments have long recognized their obligation to introduce regulations to reduce or, if possible, prevent exposure to carcinogens in the workplace. In lieu of measures that would guarantee zero exposure, governments have recognized that it is up to them to compensate for cancer caused by occupational exposure. Most workers' compensation boards do just this, using a set of guidelines to evaluate the relative toxicity of certain established carcinogens. What we need to do is establish suspected carcinogenic chemicals as *dangerous* from the outset.

Workers' right-to-know legislation exists in several states and provinces, which ought to identify hazardous chemicals and material safety information. But experts are concerned that right-to-know documents cover too few substances; for example, effluents or by-products and all pesticides are frequently exempt.

TESTING FOR TOXICITY

Testing for toxicity means proving that something is poisonous. This is often done by exposing a rat to a substance and seeing if the rat gets sick or dies. This is much easier to prove than trying to establish whether a particular poisonous substance causes cancer.

All industrialized countries share information about workplace hazards and toxic chemicals. It's no surprise that the United States is the yardstick by which Canadians measure their knowledge base—and Canada is only as safe from industrial carcinogens as its American cousin. So, how is the U.S. faring when it comes to knowledge about occupational hazards? The sad truth is: not very well at all.

There is a perception amongst the American public that because of knowledge regarding dangerous chemicals such as DDT, lead and PCBs, there is much more safety and knowledge in the workplace regarding chemical carcinogens. The U.S. Congress even passed the Toxic Substances Control Act more than 20 years ago. Yet, according to the latest data from the U.S. Environmental Defense Fund, for most of the important chemicals in American commerce, the simplest safety facts still don't exist. Even in this new century, the most basic toxicity testing results don't exist in the public record for nearly 75 percent of the top-volume chemicals in commercial use.

In the early 1980s, the U.S. National Academy of Sciences' National Research Council completed a four-year study that revealed the shocking truth: 78 percent of the chemicals in high-volume use had not been tested. When you consider that nearly 71 percent of the tested chemicals in high-volume use do not pass health hazard screening set by the Organization for Economic Cooperation and Development (OECD) Chemicals Program, this fact becomes all the more frightening. But more shocking is that we were still living in ignorance about what chemical harms may or may not be in the environment as late as the mid-1990s. In its recent report, the U.S. Environmental Defense Fund stated:

> Guinea pig status is not what Congress promised the public more than twenty years ago. Instead, it established a national policy that the risks of toxic chemicals in our environment would be identified and controlled. Ignorance, pervasive and persistent over the course of twenty years, has made that promise meaningless. (*Environmental Defense Fund Report*, 1997:6)

Getting Industry on Board

As consumers we must remind industry that we want to know the safety biographies of the products we're buying. All chemicals in high-volume use in North America ought to have been screened for at least preliminary health effects with the results publicly available for verification. A model definition of what should be included in preliminary screening tests for high-volume chemicals was developed and agreed on in 1990 by the U.S.

and the other member nations of the OECD, which includes Canada. All we've been waiting for is the industry's commitment to let the screenings begin. As consumers, we can boycott products that don't give us the information about manufacturing safety we deserve.

We already know what we don't know about industry chemicals. So the first step in protecting our workers—and ourselves—is finding out more by demanding "hazard identification," which means doing screening tests for health safety chemical by chemical. Obviously not all chemicals are toxic, but we ought to know which ones are. Here's what we should demand from any industry using chemicals:

1. Toxicity screening. These are pretty easy tests that can tell us how toxic a chemical is, and what forms of toxicity are involved. This is different from testing for cancer-causing potential. All that needs to be proven in toxicity testing is that the chemical is poisonous and "not good for us." In 1998, the U.S. EPA reported that there is no basic toxicity screening for 43 percent of the 3,000 chemicals used in the United States in quantities of one million pounds per year or more. Only 7 percent of these 3,000 chemicals have a full set of basic test data. The EPA estimated in 1998 that it would cost only 0.2 percent of the total annual sales of the top U.S. chemical companies to fill all of the basic screening data gaps for high-production volume chemicals.

2. Answers to the following about each chemical after screening. It's not enough for an industry to say, "Yep, we tested this chemical and it's safe." The following questions are based on internationally accepted criteria for toxicity screening created by the OECD Chemicals Program in 1990. If we know the answers to the following, we will know a chemical's potential to be a human health hazard.

   • What happens when you're exposed one time to chemical X (known as acute toxicity)?
   • What happens when you're exposed continuously to chemical X (known as repeated dose toxicity)?
   • What happens to a fetus's genes if a pregnant woman is exposed to chemical X (known as in vitro genetic toxicity)?
   • What happens to your own body or genes when you're exposed to chemical X (known as in vivo genetic toxicity)?
   • What happens to your reproductive organs (ovaries, breasts, breastmilk or testicles) when exposed to chemical X?
   • What happens to a developing fetus (limbs, brain, etc.) when exposed to chemical X (known as developmental toxicity/terato-

genicity)?

3. The "next steps" for each chemical tested. We should know which chemicals require no further testing; which chemicals require more testing; and which chemicals need to be controlled.

4. Open-door policies on chemical information. In chapter 2, we saw that for years the tobacco industry has been guilty of hiding its research on the dangers of tobacco from the public. We want assurance that this is not going on in other industries, and should demand that all private tests on specific chemicals that major manufacturers have performed or paid for, which to date have not been made available to the public, be made available to us. Trade secrets about a chemical should only be maintained long enough for appropriate testing to be conducted. After that, information about the chemical should be made public if it affects the public.

5. A ban on all "high-production-volume chemicals" that haven't been tested. Any chemical currently produced or imported in quantities of more than one million pounds per year should not be allowed to be in use without toxicity testing. For example, we don't know how 53 percent of high-priority chemicals affect our reproductive organs; whether 63 percent of high-priority chemicals cause cancer; whether 67 percent of high-priority chemicals affect our nervous systems or brain function; whether 86 percent of high-priority chemicals affect our immune systems; and how 90 percent of high-priority chemicals affect our children's health.

Getting Government on Board

As consumers, we should demand from our federal and state/provincial governments nothing less than what the Environmental Defense Fund demands in the face of ignorance. Writing to your federal and state departments/provincial ministries of labor and environment and demanding the following may help get the ball rolling:

- Ask for government incentives to industry to gather and disclose screening information about major chemicals and to take early steps to reduce the use of, and prevent exposures to, chemicals that have been identified as hazardous or that have not been screened.
- Demand that public disclosure on all tested chemicals be made available, and appropriately identified as safe, potentially safe (this means they are presumed safe but not absolutely proven to be safe), harmful

or potentially harmful (meaning that they are presumed harmful but not absolutely proven to be harmful).

- Demand that public disclosure on all untested chemicals be made available. A separate database should be created that lists all untested chemicals with a designation of "unknown risks" attached. Chemicals entered on this database should be given priority according to high volume usage (over a million pounds per year), so the chemicals used most get listed first until, eventually, all untested chemicals are listed.

- Demand a ban on any new, untested chemicals from entering the environment. Nothing new and untested should be used in industry until the old, untested chemicals have been tested properly. Then new chemicals can be introduced only after they've passed testing requirements. The suggestion for mutagenicity testing for new chemicals has been made in some regions. This is a red-flag test that tells us whether or not further testing for carcinogenicity is needed.

- Demand that the medical community begin compiling detailed work histories on all cancer patients so that patterns of exposure can be linked with certain cancers. This is valuable information we currently don't have.

Nobody knows whether or not a large majority of the highest-use chemicals in North America pose health hazards, or whether these chemicals are actually under control. We really don't know what we're likely to breathe or drink or house in our bodies. And we don't know what is being released from industrial facilities into our backyards, streets, forests and streams.

A lot of what you've read in this chapter has likely disturbed you. But knowing what we don't know is the first step in lobbying for more information so that future generations have better ways to protect themselves, which is what primary prevention of cancer is all about. I'm afraid the news gets worse as you read on, but the suggestions for improving the state of the earth get better. So take heart by taking charge! Your children will thank you.

Many chemicals are under suspicion because they have been proven to cause cancer in animals but have not yet been conclusively shown to cause human cancer. The list is quite long. Here are some of the more common ones:

> Cadmium
> Carbon Tetrachloride
> Chloroform

Dibromochlorpropane (DBCP)
Diesel exhaust
Ethylene Theourea
Formaldehyde
Isocyanates

The "Least-Wanted List"
Known Cancer Agents

There is sufficient evidence to prove these substances cause cancer in humans. This is a partial list.

Chemical	Type of Cancer
Acrylonitrile	Lung
4-Aminobiphenyl	Urinary bladder
Arsenic	Lung, skin
Asbestos	Lung, several others
Benzene	Leukemia (white blood cells)
Benzidine	Urinary bladder
Beryllium	Lung
Bis-chloromethyl ether (BCME)	Lung
Chloromethyl methyl ether	Lung
Chromates, most types	Lung, larynx, nasal cavity
Coal Tar	Lung, skin, bladder
Ethylene oxide	Lymphatic, blood
Metalworking Fluids	Skin, larynx, rectum, stomach, esophagus, colon, bladder, sinonasal, lung, prostate, pancreas
Mustard Gas	Lung
2-Naphthylamine	Urinary bladder
Nickel and its compounds	Lung, nasal cavity
Polycyclic Aromatic Hydrocarbons (a.k.a. PAHs, poly nuclera aromatics or PNAs—includes coke oven emissions, soot and various kinds of smoke)	Lung, several others
Radon	Lung
Tobacco Smoke—Secondhand Smokers	Lung, mouth, larynx, lips, throat, bladder, kidney, pancreas
Vinyl Chloride	Liver, brain, lymphatic, blood
Wood Dusts (Limited types)	Nasal cavity, possibly others

Kepone
MOCA (a.k.a. curene or methylene-bis-chloroaniline)
Nitrosamines
PCBs (poly chlorinated biphenyls)
Perchloroethylene ("Perc")
Trichloroethylene (TCE)
Tris 2, 3 dibromoppropyl phosphate ("Tris")
Vinyl Bromide

Source: The Canadian Autoworkers Health and Safety Department. Cancer in Your Workplace: A Manual for Worker Investigators. *1999:28-29.*

Scenes of the Crime
Possible High-Risk Jobs

These can involve exposure to known animal or human carcinogens.

Job	Carcinogen
Brake-shoe manufacture	Asbestos
Pipefitting	Asbestos
Selected welding and grinding jobs	Beryllium, Chromium, Cadmium, Nickel, Stainless steel (chrome and nickel)
Forming and curing certain plastics	Acrylonitrile, MOCA (a.k.a. curene or methylene-bis-chloroaniline), Formaldehyde, Styrene
Degreasing and cold cleaning with chlorinated solvents	Trichloroethylene
Foundry core-making	Formaldehyde
Metalworking-engine plants, components plants, parts plants, aerospace, machine shops	Metalworking fluids
Mining-smelting and milling	Diesel exhaust, oil mists, radon gas, arsenic, PAHs, EMFs (electro magnetic fields)

Source: The Canadian Autoworkers Health and Safety Department. Cancer in Your Workplace: A Manual for Worker Investigators. 1999:30

Workplaces under Investigation
These are under suspicion because of preliminary cancer studies. More work is needed to pin down specific jobs or chemicals.

- Foundry work, especially core-making and exposure to mould burn-off.
- Machining operations with oil and coolant mist (e.g., bearing plants, engine plants).
- Wood model and pattern making.
- Motor-vehicle-assembly plants.
- Plating and die-casting operations.
- Smelters—PAHs, EMFs, nickel

Jobs with Special Considerations

- Processes with oil smoke such as forging operations, heat treat, hot die work. Many of these jobs involve exposure to various polycyclic aromatic hydrocarbons (PAHs), some of which are known to cause human cancer. Adequate air measurements or mortality studies have not been done in most cases.
- Work around diesel exhaust. Diesel particulate can carry various PAH chemicals deep into the lung. It is known that diesel exhaust can cause serious damage to bacteria. Excess cancers have been seen among locomotive engineers and miners.
- Fiber glass fabrication. Dust from small-diameter fiber glass is a cancer hazard, depending on the size and shape of the glass fiber.
- Work with metalworking fluids.

Scientific studies have shown that workers in a variety of industries are at high cancer risk. The specific types of cancer vary and the chemicals responsible are not fully established in all cases:

Rubber industry workers—nitrosamines, NDMA (N-
                    nitrosodimethylamine)
Uranium miners—radon gas
Nickel smelting workers—nickel
Petroleum refinery workers—benzene
Aluminum smelter workers—EMFs, PAHs
Copper smelting workers—arsenic
Roofers—coal tar, PAHs
Hematitie miners
Leather and shoe workers—chromates
Printing press workers—solvents
Hospital operating room personnel—ethylene oxide
Wood products workers—pentachlorophenol, creosote
                    reosote, arsenic, chromium
                    (wood preservatives)
Chemical dye manufacturers—benzidines

Source: The Canadian Autoworkers Health and Safety Department. Cancer in Your Workplace: A Manual for Worker Investigators. 1999:31.

8
EARTH, WIND AND FIRE

One of the most unsettling experiences of my life was watching a *Sesame Street* vignette called "Where does rain come from?" As my 4-year-old niece sat with her apple juice, fascinated by the story of clouds, air condensation and all the other interesting facts behind what makes rain, all I could think of was how interconnected everything was, and how airborne contaminants could easily poison our water, and vice versa. If you know where rain comes from, you know how dangerous airborne contaminants are to our health. By taking a closer look at the accumulation of toxic substances in our air, water and food supply, we can begin to explore what has been increasingly recognized as a major threat to human health.

ENVIRONMENTAL CARCINOGENS

In 1962, environmentalist Rachel Carson wrote a book called *Silent Spring*, which essentially said: wake up and smell the chemicals; wildlife and humans are dying from exposure to pesticides and pollutants. Carson was denounced by industry and medical leaders as hysterical; she died of breast cancer in 1964. Today, many renowned scientists in both the environmental and medical research community are concluding that maverick Rachel Carson was right all along. Dr. Theo Colborne, senior scientist at the World Wildlife Fund and co-author of *Our Stolen Future* (1996), and Dr. Sandra Steingraber, whose book, *Living Downstream: An Ecologist Looks At Cancer and The Environment* (1997) is being seen as this generation's *Silent Spring*, have taken up Carson's cause. Dr. Steingraber put it best at a lecture she gave in 1997 at the World Conference on Breast Cancer in Kingston: "Science likes to prove the same thing over and over again before it says that something is fact. And that's usually a good thing. But sometimes calling for more research is the grandfather excuse for doing nothing." This sentiment is echoed by the International Joint Commission on the Great Lakes: "Scientific arguments and their lack of absolute proof can also be used as an excuse for inaction. The phrase 'good science' has been used to block change through demands for more rigorous proof." (Eighth Biennial Report On Great Lakes Water Quality, 1996, p. 17). Indeed, had we waited for clear scientific proof that cigarettes cause lung cancer, we'd still be waiting for that surgeon general's warning.

The term "environmental carcinogens" refers to cancer-causing agents that are in our environment: the air, soil and water. So whatever comes into contact with this air, soil and water can become contaminated. The implications for our food chain are clear—plants and animals nourished by contaminated soil and water become contaminated. By using the province of Ontario as a test case for large urban centers, we can glimpse the toxic state of affairs in other parts of North America.

In October 1993, the Ontario Ministry of Environment and Energy released a report called "Candidate Substances for Bans, Phase-Outs and Reductions." There were two parts to the report, each part containing a list of dangerous substances. The primary list identified 20 substances either present in, or discharged into, the Ontario environment. All of these substances were considered inherently hazardous due to their persistence in water, sediment, air or soil, their tendency to accumulate in the environment and their toxicity. All in all, 1,000 substances were evaluated. Fifteen of the substances on the primary list were classified as Group 1 or Group 2 carcinogens. These classifications were based on criteria set out by the World Health Organization's International Agency for Research on Cancer (IARC). The IARC's list contains pretty much the same information as a similar list periodically updated by the U.S. Environmental Protection Agency.

Another list of persistent toxic substances, this one put together by the Accelerated Reduction/Elimination of Toxins (ARET) project, contained over 70 identified or suspected carcinogens. Carcinogens on ARET's A-1 list (those that met or exceeded ARET's criteria for toxicity, accumulation and persistence) include: all polychlorinated biphenyls; polycyclic aromatic hydrocarbons (PAHs); 1,8-dinitro-pyrene; and five types of chlorinated organics, also called organochorines. The substances on all these lists are in the air, the soil and the water around us. See the IARC tables at the end of this chapter for a complete list (or what we know so far).

What Are We Breathing?

We are exposed to countless known or suspected carcinogens every day. Present in our air, our water, our soil and consequently our food, these contaminants are impossible to avoid. Our skin absorbs them, our lungs inhale them, and we ingest them just about every time we eat. A study conducted by the City of Toronto Health Department identified 160 trace compounds present in Toronto air. That number included 4 human carcinogens and another 27 suspected carcinogens. And while the levels of air toxins in Toronto were still within provincial air quality standards, many of the substances exceeded the levels thought to increase the risk of cancer. If you live in a large urban center, a similar study will probably reveal the same results in your local area.

A two-year study near Detroit, Michigan (in Windsor, Ontario) was undertaken in response to concerns that air pollution was drifting across the Canada–U.S. border. The community was worried about the quality of both outdoor and indoor air. And for good reason. Forty air pollutants were investigated, ten of which have been known to cause risks to human health in the long term. Five of these ten pollutants were found to be present in high concentrations in both indoor and outdoor air; benzene, 1,3-butadiene and chromium (VI) raised cancer risks via indoor and outdoor air, while cadmium, carbon tetrachloride, 1,4-dichlorobenzene, formaldehyde and PAHs increased cancer risk via indoor air.

Car exhaust

Car exhaust (known as vehicle emissions) is considered to be among the primary sources of carcinogens in the air supply of many Western countries. Car exhaust powered by fossil fuels contains a number of suspected carcinogens, including benzene and polycyclic aromatic hydrocarbons.

What Are We Ingesting?

The most serious hazards affecting our food are what are called persistent toxic substances. These are so named because they are, well, *persistent*. They remain in the biophysical environment for long periods of time and become widely dispersed, establishing themselves in the plants and animals (including humans!) that ingest them as part of the food chain. Sadly, the ecosystem is incapable of breaking down many of these substances. Because they are not naturally occurring chemicals (with their own built-in metabolic pathways for detoxifying themselves), the ecosystem has no way to absorb them. In fact, many of these chemicals have been developed *because* they are not readily metabolized and detoxified! They stick around and by so doing, cause any number of adverse health effects, including cancer in humans and animals.

We can be pretty certain that persistent toxic substances in our water and soil have entered our food chain. In a pilot study of the different ways human beings are exposed to toxic chemicals in the Great Lakes Basin, it was estimated that about 85 percent of toxic exposure that isn't work-related comes from food products. A follow-up study investigating a larger sample of food products found lower residue levels of organochlorines. But this particular study concluded that 95 percent of our exposure to one group of contaminants (polychlorinated dibenzo-p-dioxins and polychlorinated dibenzofurans) comes from the food we eat. The fact that these substances are being absorbed into our food chain is cause for alarm. It is one of the most compelling reasons we have for "sunsetting" (meaning, "ridding within a certain timetable") persistent toxic substances that are known or suspected carcinogens.

Organochlorines
Certain classes of persistent toxic chemicals are particularly dangerous. To curtail the risks associated with them, it may make sense to deal with these chemicals as a class or group, instead of addressing them one at a time. Organochlorines are a case in point.

Organochlorines make up a class of chemicals created by the combination of chlorine and various organic compounds. They include chemicals like DDT, PCBs, dioxin, chlordane and hexachlorobenzene. Many of these substances are also considered animal carcinogens, and are thought to be possible human carcinogens. Some organochlorines can impair our immune systems or mimic estrogen and, most serious of all, cause our bodies to grow tumors.

Organochlorines get into the soil, giving them a direct route into the food chain—which is how they get into human beings. Trace residues of organochlorines have shown up in the fatty tissues of birds, animals and humans. They have also been found in human breast milk.

Thankfully, some chlorinated organics, including PCBs and DDT, have been banned, but others continue to be used in pesticides. Organochlorines are also used in the making of PVC (polyvinyl chloride) plastics, and are produced in the bleaching process at pulp and paper mills and the incineration process of chlorine-containing products, such as yogurt containers and plastic bags.

Radioactivity

Our collective fears around radiation exposure have escalated in recent years following events like the Chernobyl nuclear accident in 1986. Exposure to hazardous levels of radiation has long been recognized as a cause of leukemia and other cancers, particularly thyroid cancer, as a result of radioactive iodine, a substance that is emitted in the fallout caused by nuclear explosions.

The Chernobyl accident released 40 million curies of radioactive iodine into the atmosphere, exposing millions of people to excessive levels of radioactive iodine. People living within 30 kilometres of the accident inhaled the radioactive iodine, and people living outside this radius were exposed to the substance. The incidence of thyroid cancer in children in Belarus, Russia and the Ukraine appears to have increased twentyfold as a result of exposure. A Ukraine study reports that between 1981 and 1985, the number of new cases of thyroid cancer in children up to age 14 totalled 25. But between 1986 and 1994, the number of new cases of thyroid cancer in this age group totalled 210, peaking in 1992 and 1993.

In the United States, a National Cancer Institute study published in 1997 looked at the health effects of radioactive fallout released at a Nevada nuclear test site between 1951 and 1958. The study concludes that people living in the midwestern regions of North America might be more at risk for thyroid cancer, particularly if they were children when the testing was conducted. The North Dakota State Health Department reported in 1994 that the incidence of thyroid cancer in that state had doubled from 5 percent to 10 percent, an increase that was attributed to radioactive iodine fallout. Furthermore, the U.S. Energy Research Foundation concludes that there may be thousands of North Americans who ingested milk contaminated by this fallout, and who are at greater risk for thyroid cancer. The Oak Ridge Health Agreement Steering Panel reports that, of women born in 1952, those in the midwestern United States who drank milk contaminated by the test fallout are more likely to develop thyroid cancer in their lifetime than are women who were born in the northeastern states.

Evidence has been collected from the studies of people with medical exposures to high doses of radiation, and from the studies of atomic bomb survivors in Japan that indicate that the improper management, storage and disposal of nuclear waste can produce harmful effects (i.e., cancer) in people who live and work close to the waste products.

Tritium

Tritium, a radioactive isotope of hydrogen, is a by-product of nuclear reactor operations. It cannot be removed from drinking water with conventional water treatment systems. The EPA in the United States classifies tritium as a human carcinogen. There is some evidence that elevated levels of tritium in Ontario drinking water may be a result of emissions from nuclear facilities in Pickering and Darlington. In a 1991 study, Ontario Hydro revealed that tritium concentrations in drinking water taken from Lake Ontario at the Ajax, Whitby, Oshawa, Scarborough and Toronto treatment plants were higher than the Lake Ontario average. Ontario Hydro blamed the increase on emissions from the Pickering and Darlington nuclear generating stations.

In 1994, the Advisory Committee on Environmental Standards recommended that the Ontario Drinking Water Objective significantly reduce the levels of tritium within five years. To date, the Ontario government has not acted on this recommendation. Because we're still uncertain of the potential harms caused by this substance, we can only hope that initiatives like this one will eliminate it from our drinking water.

HOW DO WE KNOW THESE SUBSTANCES ARE DANGEROUS?

We know what we're breathing and ingesting is probably dangerous based on an accumulating body of scientific evidence, which includes:

- Studies, like those done on the emission of diesel exhaust, that have identified air pollution as a cause of lung cancer. Other studies have found high rates of lung cancer among people living near large petrochemical plants. One Canadian study identified a link between sulphur dioxide and ground-level ozone emissions and the incidence of breast and colon cancer.
- Ecological studies, like those that prove proximity to a hazardous waste site can increase the risk of breast and other cancers.
- Studies conducted on animals that show a positive correlation between organochlorines and breast cancer. A possible link also exists between breast cancer and exposure to xeno-estrogens, estrogen-like substances released into the environment as pesticides or industrial chemicals, which accumulate in body fat. The more estrogen women are exposed to in their lifetimes, the greater their risk of breast cancer. However, evidence of the association between organochlorines (often made up of xeno-estrogens) and breast cancer is inconclusive.

- Studies that identify exposure to hazardous levels of radiation as a cause of leukemia. There is also a suspected association between leukemia and exposure to electromagnetic fields.
- Results of a metanalysis (a review of other studies) that demonstrated the danger of water disinfection by-products like chlorinated organics (formed when chlorine meets naturally occurring humic and fulvic acids). These toxins may be responsible for some 10,000 bladder and rectal cancer deaths in the United States each year.

Limitations of Science

As stated earlier, the problem with proving that all of these environmental hazards are affecting our health is that we can't prove it beyond a reasonable doubt. We suspect but can't absolutely prove, which is why it's so hard to get government and industry to take action to eliminate environmental contaminants. Showing that a substance is toxic is different than linking that toxic substance to negative human health effects. Business and government like to act based on conclusive evidence provided by science. We will never be able to provide that proof because *science* is still unsure about certain untested or poorly tested environmental contaminants. What can we do? We have to demand that to protect our health, the government should never assume that a chemical is safe until it is proven to be safe.

Why is the science so unreliable? There are limits to the scientific methods used to do these studies. There's no way to control a study looking at the effects of environmental toxins on human health because:

1. There are too many variables. We are exposed to a wide variety of environmental pollutants every day. Often, it is a combination of many substances that creates risk. These combinations vary according to where we live, our economic status, our lifestyle and our work. Trying to figure out which parts of each combination of exposures are attributable to pollution in the environment can be very difficult.

2. We can't "control" whole populations for a study. For many substances, especially those that have been very widely dispersed in the environment, control groups (those that haven't been exposed and can, therefore, act as a point of reference) are impossible to find. It's also difficult to find and assess groups of people with different levels of exposure because these substances are everywhere. Most human populations, for example, now carry detectable levels of suspected carcinogens (e.g.,

DDT, PCBs) in their body fat.

3. We need to study things for a long time. The length of time required for accurate results hinders our attempts to put numbers to the cancer/pollution association. Often, only small groups of people have experienced high levels of exposure. Or, we must wait years to confirm a cancer diagnosis. Sometimes, too, subjects withdraw from a study, or the study is abandoned due to high costs.

4. Too many toxins to study. We have yet to accumulate toxicological data on some 80 percent of the 45,000–100,000 chemicals in common use today. Data on chronic effects are especially limited. However, more than 1,000 chemicals (or combinations of chemicals) have been evaluated by the IARC (see the material at the end of this chapter), and only 30 of them have been found to be carcinogenic. Another 20 are classified as probably carcinogenic to humans and 93 as possibly carcinogenic. It is important to remember that much evidence is needed to identify a substance as carcinogenic. Many chemicals have been identified as "probable" or "possible" carcinogens simply because we lack the proof to call them "known." On the brighter side, many substances are selected for assessment by the IARC based on preliminary evidence that they are carcinogenic; this evidence is only suggestive. Many of the untested substances may not be carcinogenic at all.

5. Existing data is still being attacked. Not all scientists agree with the studies to date, and many insist they are not proof of anything. Interpretations of data differ for a number of reasons: the dose-level administered in animal testing is often inconsistent; it's difficult to draw conclusions for one species based on the results from testing on another, completely different species; and the models used and assumptions made during testing often don't translate into human risk factor at the other end of the process.

The bottom line is that the "solid proof" model is unworkable when dealing with environmental carcinogens and should be abandoned in favor of new approaches outlined next.

The Weight of Evidence Approach

Since we have yet to see any real proof as defined by conventional science of the health risks caused by environmental toxins, we need to work with what we have. That means adopting a "weight of evidence" approach to assessing risk, combining results from different fields of study, including wildlife observations and laboratory testing.

That doesn't mean we should halt future research, but rather, we shouldn't wait for any further research before beginning to act on what we know now. For instance, estimates of the proportion of cancers caused by environmental carcinogens vary from 2 to 20 percent. It's hard to come up with exact numbers since most of them are based on a combination of daily and workplace exposures. As consumers, we should be informed by science, but our governments have a responsibility to be informed of our values as consumers and citizens, which means they must err on the side of caution.

WHAT ARE THE HEALTH RISKS?

In her book, *Living Downstream*, Dr. Sandra Steingraber notes that beluga whales in the polluted St. Lawrence River have high rates of bladder, stomach, intestinal, salivary gland, breast and ovarian cancers. Meanwhile, beluga whales in the Atlantic Ocean are cancer free. Steingraber herself was diagnosed with bladder cancer at the age of 20. She quotes conservationist Leone Pippard:

> Tell me, does the St. Lawrence beluga drink too much alcohol and does the St. Lawrence beluga smoke too much and does the St. Lawrence beluga have a bad diet? Is that why the beluga whales are ill? Do you think you are somehow immune and that it's only the beluga whale that is being affected? (Steingraber, Sandra. *Living Downstream*. Addison-Wesley, 1997:139.)

Persistent, bioconcentrating toxic substances, meaning toxic substances that live in human and animal fat or settle onto plants, have been linked to all manner of disease and disorder in humans and animals. These toxins can affect everything from reproductive health and immune system functions to behavior and respiratory systems. For example, ground-level ozone, which forms when car exhaust and industry gases interact with the sunlight, is known to cause decreased lung capabilities and other respiratory problems.

Some of the most disturbing evidence documenting the harmful effects of environmental pollutants comes from wildlife studies conducted in areas close to heavy industrial activity. Wildlife exposed to industrial chemicals, for example, show abnormally high numbers of birth defects and reproductive disorders. This phenomenon is almost certainly caused by a sort of "confusion" of natural, biological processes. Environmental contaminants in this case mimic the effect of naturally occurring hormones, disrupting the animal's natural life functions.

What can our governments do about this?
Ideally, our governments ought to act on many of the following recommendations, which are based on previous proposals by provincial, national and international bodies. Some of these recommendations address the problem of persistent toxic chemicals in general; others deal separately with specific known or suspected carcinogens. In some cases, dealing with groups of substances at a time (like those at work in incinerators, landfills or vehicle emis-

Environmental Estrogens

Environmental scientists have begun to notice that several wildlife species are experiencing hermaphroditic traits. In the Florida swamplands, alligators are simply not breeding. A concerned research team from the University of Florida went into the swamps to find out why. These researchers pulled male alligators out of the water to examine their genitals. The majority of male alligators they found were sterile as a result of either non-developed or abnormally shaped penises. A chemical spill in nearby waters was found to be the culprit, which was having an "estrogenic effect" on the alligators' natural habitat.

Meanwhile, 2,300 kilometers north in a Canadian creek on Lake Superior, scientists found that fish living in waters close to a pulp mill, which contained certain chemicals with estrogenic effects, were now complete hermaphrodites. The male fish in these waters had developed ovaries and were sterile; the female fish had exaggerated ovaries. In other contaminated waters, fish had actually exploded from thyroid hormone overactivity.

Researchers in Sweden and the United Kingdom have been concerned since the late 1980s over a dramatic increase in male infertility in their countries, while there is an increased incidence of male infants being born with cryptorchidism, a condition in which the testicles do not descend into the scrotum, but remain undescended inside the abdomen. One study found that there has indeed been a huge decrease over the last 50 years in the quality of human semen. (A recent study measuring sperm quality in New York City contradicted these findings.) There has also been a huge increase in the incidence of testicular and prostate cancers. In Britain, testicular cancer incidence has tripled over the last 50 years; it is now the most common cancer in young men under 30. In Denmark, there has been a 400 percent increase in testicular cancer. As for prostate cancer, its incidence has doubled over the last decade. These male reproductive problems have been linked to environmental estrogens, too.

The scientific literature is slowly becoming saturated with findings linking one organic chemical after another to reproductive cancers and "endocrine disruption" in both wildlife and humans. Every study, from all corners of the world, is reaching the same conclusion: organic chemicals are transforming into environmental estrogens. And they're everywhere. Organic chemicals are in the air we breathe from numerous air pollutants; in the food preservatives used in numerous canned and packaged goods; and in the pesticides used on fresh produce. These chemicals then contaminate the water and soil, which contaminate the entire human food chain.

Some suggest that environmental estrogens are "feminizing" the planet. Some suggest that women are being overloaded with estrogen, which may be associated with the rise of estrogen-dependent cancers, such as ovarian and breast cancer, as well as estrogen-related conditions, such as endometriosis (an estrogenic condition where pieces of the uterine lining grow outside the uterus and can block the fallopian tubes) and fibroids. Estrogen pollutants are also thought to accumulate in fatty tissues (meaning they are stored in fat). Since women generally carry more body fat than men, women may be accumulating more of these toxins. Some studies have already found that women with breast cancer tend to have higher concentrations of the organochlorines DDT, DDE or PCBs in their fat tissue. In fact, elevated levels of DDE in the blood have been directly linked to a fourfold increase of breast cancer in the United States. We already know that dioxins, also organocholorines, are associated with endometriosis.

Some suggest that the picture is equally dismal for men, many of whom are not only becoming slowly sterilized by this phenomenon, but are also developing reproductive cancers. Several prominent scientists have gone on record to say that this problem is the environmental priority of the twenty-first century!

On the flip side, many doctors point out that in the Western world, there has also been a huge increase in the "fatness" of the population. This also increases the level of estrogen produced by our bodies.

sions) is a better strategy. Controlling the level of toxic chemicals in our air, water, soil and food supply can only have a positive effect on the control of specific known or suspected carcinogens.

Changing the Standards of Proof

Stopping Cancer at the Source

One of the most important changes governments can make to protect public health is to change their standards of proof. Right now, governments like conclusive proof that a chemical or substance is toxic or harmful before they ban it. This isn't realistic. Instead, governments ought to withhold approval of chemicals for use until there is conclusive proof that they are safe. Erring on the side of caution is the best policy. In other words, chemicals should be "suspected carcinogens" until they are proven to be non-carcinogenic. This is especially important for new substances.

This policy won't help reduce the amount of persistent toxic substances already in use, but it will, at least, prevent more from being added to the environment. That said, we can certainly ban the import of persistent toxic substances. (There are no "air borders," of course, but we can ban certain produce known to be sprayed with certain pesticides, and so forth.)

Sunsetting

Sunsetting is a step-by-step process that aims to restrict, phase-out and one day ban the production, generation, use, transport, storage, discharge and disposal of a persistent toxic substance. Sunsetting involves two things:

1. It targets the chemical and the manufacturing and production processes associated with that chemical.
2. It looks at ways of eliminating the substance within realistic parameters.

Reducing the Health Risks

Instead of ignoring the health risks associated with environment contaminants the population is facing, governments should face them and deal with them. Some ways to deal with them include:

- Making the pollution prevention agencies work with industrial policy authorities so that the technology of business and the technology of research share some common ground.
- Adopting the rigorous standards for controlling environmental carcinogens developed by Organization for Economic Cooperation and Development (OECD) member nations.
- Making a list of what's toxic, suspected to be toxic and definitely not toxic so everyone knows. The Ontario Ministry of Environment and Energy's "Candidate Substances for Bans, Phase-Outs or Reductions" is a good example of this.
- Banning organochlorines. Knowing what we do about organochlorines,

how can we still allow them into our atmosphere? Many contend that there are chlorine compounds that can be used safely. Chlorine has a preventive side, too. It is commonly used for water purification, needle sterilization and chlorinated pharmaceutical production. But perhaps those benefits can be found using a different process or non-carcinogenic chemical. Perhaps we need to deal with organochlorines as a class of toxic chemicals, and sunset them accordingly. In establishing timetables for sunsetting, then, we may want to think about first banning those organochlorines that are themselves carcinogenic, or those that have been known to introduce carcinogens into the environment.

Banning All Carcinogenic Pesticides

There are non-carcinogenic pesticides that we can use these days. The use of suspected carcinogenic pesticides has contaminated both our environment and our food chain. A number of pesticides that are known animal and suspected human carcinogens are actually registered as legal for use. Contamination occurs differently than you might think. It's not that the food we eat contains detectable residues of harmful organochlorines because it's been sprayed with pesticides, but rather that these substances have started to accumulate in our surface water, groundwater, sediment, soil and air. These substances are absorbed into the food as it grows, at the cell level. It is this concentration within the food *chain* of bioaccumulative substances that poses the greatest threat to human health.

It's estimated that billions of gallons of toxic pesticides have been released into an unsuspecting environment. Since these chemicals are resistant to breaking down, as mentioned above, they're spread around the world through the air and water, exposing us to these poisons in our food, groundwater, surface water and air. According to a 1992 Greenpeace report on chlorine and human health, no industrial organochlorines are known to be non-toxic.

Approximately 1,300 farm wells in Ontario were tested for pesticide residues in the winter of 1991–92, and retested the following summer. Eight percent of the wells in winter and 12 percent of the wells in summer showed detectable levels of pesticide residues. Two wells showed levels higher than the Interim Maximum Acceptable Concentration (IMAC) values of 5 parts per billion, a finding that is thought to be the result of a nearby chemical spill.

The consumption of certain popular food products containing the residues of 28 different pesticides has been blamed on some 20,000 excess cancer deaths in the United States each year. This is a controversial estimate, however, and many believe it should be used only in relation to preventive dietary measures (if you eat your fruits and veggies, their protective factor will overwhelm the cancer-causing hazards of pesticide residues in foods).

To further address cancer risks associated with exposure to pesticides, experts recommend:

- Developing and applying alternative, non-chemical pest-control methods, such as those used by organic growers.
- Sunsetting the following chemicals, which meet IARC/USEPA (U.S. Environmental Protection Agency) criteria for known or suspected carcinogens, still registered for use across North America: Group 2A (see p. 140) (probable human carcinogens): ethylene oxide (insecticide, fungicide), formaldehyde (antimicrobial), creosote (wood preservative); Group 2B (possible human carcinogens): amitrole (herbicide), atrazine (herbicide), dichlorvos (insecticide), hexachlorocyclo-hexanes (lindane–gamma-HCH, insecticide, acaricide), pentachlorophenol (wood preservative), sodium ortho-phenylphenate (antimicrobial).

Reducing Radiation Risks

In order to control the cancer risks associated with hazardous levels of radiation, and to start identifying where unrecognized hazards from exposure might occur, experts recommend:

- Developing an inventory of sources of radioactive nuclides in Canada and the United States.
- Investigating how radioactive substances travel through the food chain.
- Imposing "chemical control rules" for suspected radioactive contaminants, which would result in more stringent standards.
- Studying radioactive emissions from energy production plants.
- Investigating ways of phasing out these materials wherever an increased cancer risk is found.

Reducing Car Exhaust

Car exhaust is making us sick. Cancer is just one of many health risks linked to motor vehicle emissions today.

Ground-level ozone is created when volatile organic compounds meet nitrogen oxides (found in emissions from burning fossil fuels), and has been associated with lung diseases and other respiratory problems. Worst of all, car exhaust leads to "earth sickness" because it is the ground-level ozone from motor vehicle emissions that causes both global warming and acid rain. Put the two together, and the damage to the ecosystem (not to mention our health!) may be irreparable.

To reduce car exhaust from our lives, here are some steps many governments are already taking:

- Decrease emissions from all sources. That includes from cars, trucks and motorcycles as well as two-stroke engines (like lawn mowers, chainsaws, minibikes, motorboats and some mopeds) that emit benzene and PAHs.
- Test vehicles regularly for hazardous levels of emissions. (Ontario has just started to do this; California is already seeing huge improvements in its air quality through this measure.)
- Start gasoline vapor recovery programs at all fuel transfer facilities and gas stations to reduce unwanted benzene emissions. (This is in place in several areas across North America; California was one of the first to implement it and is seeing the positive results.)
- Support research on the development of alternative, environmentally friendly fuels (like hydrogen) that reduce the overall impact on the environment.
- Encourage people to change the way they get to work (for example, walking, cycling, public transit).
- Subsidize less polluting forms of travel. This could mean anything from decreased public transit fares to newer, more accessible bicycle lanes. The point is to discourage urban sprawl and subsidize public transit.
- Engage in judicious urban planning so that more people can afford to live close to where they work and shop (big box stores are the wrong way to go!).

"But I love my car!"

Let's face it, if you're like me, you may love your car, too. But maybe we can learn to love cars that run on cleaner fuel, or learn to drive partway to our destination, incorporating nice long walks or bicycling into some of the journey. Plus, we don't have to drive to places that are, in fact, within walking distance.

Creating New Jobs Through Alternative Safe Substances

Governments can get industry on board by creating incentives for it to come up with alternatives to the toxic substances now in use. If we can build atomic bombs and come up with ways to destroy the earth, surely we can come up with ways to protect it by creating new, environmentally sustainable products, industries and technologies. This would reduce our cost of living rather than increase it. And we'd gain back planetary health for future generations.

Many European countries, for example, are developing feasible, cost-effective alternatives to some of the toxic substance currently used and produced in North America. Since the whole world is concerned, new alternatives could mean big bucks for the manufacturers or creators of those alternatives. North American governments ought to look at environmentally friendly initiatives as "job creation" rather than "job destruction" initiatives.

That said, by eliminating many of these persistent toxic substances, jobs will be affected. Therefore, our governments can:

- Develop transition plans to aid those who will be adversely affected by the elimination of the use and production of these substances.
- Create a taxation scheme whereby taxes are increased in small increments to provide economic incentives for the reduction of toxic emissions during the phase-out period.
- Develop a fund from those tax revenues to help in the transition to a less toxic industrial society. The funds could be used to explore and demonstrate economically viable alternatives and, again, to aid those workers who have lost their jobs as a result of the transition.

Supporting Public Education Initiatives

The public has a right to know what's going on. Educational programs (including public reports on health and the environment) would be better off addressing the spectrum of issues stemming from environmental health concerns, rather than focusing specifically on cancer. To increase public awareness of environmental health issues, governments can:

- Continue to develop environmental health sciences programs at the grade school level, teaching students how environmental science works, and how relationships between health and the environment work. Industry can help fund special programs in this area, too.
- Encourage university-age students to go into the environmental sciences so they can help solve tomorrow what we can't solve today.
- Support non-governmental groups and organizations in their efforts to educate the public and to develop community action plans.
- Support community action plans that encourage prevention.
- Support intersectoral (meaning, multiple industries coming together) activities on environment and health.

HOW CAN WE HELP OURSELVES?

The first thing we can do to help ourselves is to send the message to our governments and industries that we can't afford to wait for the science. Because we don't yet know the extent to which environmental contaminants contribute to cancer, public health and health promotion experts agree that the only prudent approach to safeguarding the health of the general public is to be precautionary, and wait until research makes us sure. In other words, we should presume the guilt of a potentially toxic substance before we judge it to be innocent. Don't release it into the atmosphere until it's proven safe. This is the "science will follow" versus "no danger yet" approach. For now, we ought to demand policies that protect the public from any known or suspected human and animal carcinogens, as no dose of a carcinogen can be considered a safe dose.

Finding Out the Facts

Consumers have a right to know the following:

- Known and suspected environmental carcinogens.
- The cancers associated with each environmental carcinogen.
- What science can prove and what it can't prove (as mentioned earlier, it's difficult to absolutely prove certain links because of the way we are trained to research, and because sometimes there are just too many variables involved).
- The other health risks (i.e., reproductive disorders) posed by environmental carcinogens.
- Strategies already in place for reducing or, where possible, eliminating exposure to environmental carcinogens.

Limiting Your Exposure

Right now, the only hope we have of eliminating environmental toxins is through consumer lobbying. The best place to start the environmental cleanup is in your kitchen. Your weekly groceries probably contain residues from pesticides and other organochlorines (on store-bought fruits and vegetables), hormones in meat products, as well as a number of "extras" you may not have bargained for, which were fed to your meat when it was still alive. These include feed additives, antibiotics and tranquilizers. Meanwhile, anything packaged will most likely contain dyes and flavors from a variety of chemical concoctions.

Stopping Cancer at the Source

Airborne contaminants, waste and spills affect the water and soil, which affect everything we ingest. When one species becomes unable to reproduce, we could lose not just that species but all those that depend on it, thus disrupting the food chain. Cleaning up the food chain is all part of creating a healthy, contaminant-free diet for ourselves. So make the following grocery list before your next shopping trip:

- You can find out what your produce has eaten, and whether it was injected with anything by contacting the Canadian Food Inspection Agency at *www.cfia-acia.agr.ca* or the U.S. National Food Safety Database at *www.foodsafety.org*.
- You can find out what waters your fish has swum in by contacting the above organizations.
- You can find out what your produce was sprayed with by contacting the above organizations.
- You can find "safe food" that is organically grown or raised through a number of natural produce supermarkets or get in touch with the Organic Trade Association (serving both Canada and the United States) at *www.ota.com*.

You can find out more about your supermarket's buying habits when it comes to produce by contacting your supermarket's head office.

Since the word "consumer" comes from the word "consume"—to eat—becoming vigilant about our groceries is the only way to help change the food industry. Customers are incredibly powerful to any company. In the 1980s, it was the "vigilant consumer" who helped to make manufacturers more green-friendly and value-conscious. In many instances, the sheer volume of customer complaints and customer letters has completely changed not only certain companies' habits and policies, but also an entire industry. If enough customers boycott products and protest manufacturing or agricultural practices, the companies will change. Start lobbying for change, and bring new meaning to the adage "The customer is always right!"

Read any good labels lately?
Worried about the plastic that lines certain canned goods? Demand labeling that identifies the organic chemicals used to make that plastic. Worried about the plastics used in various cosmetics, detergents and spermicides? Then write letters to manufacturers; call 800 numbers; start a newsgroup on the Internet; lobby; protest; boycott products to help change standards. Don't be afraid to write letters to the editors of daily newspapers or call for press conferences on various labeling, packaging or ingredient issues that

concern you. What exactly is plastic wrap made out of anyway? You have a right to know. What was this spinach sprayed with? You have a right to a label that reads: "This produce sprayed with endosulfan." To date, the chemical ingredients that make up plastic products are kept from the consumer because they're considered trade secrets. This is unacceptable. As consumers, we must use our collective voice to help get labeling details on the containers that house our produce, as well as on our meat and dairy products. Perhaps Faith Popcorn, author of *The Popcorn Report*, put it best when she predicted that by 2010:

> Labels will become more important than ever before. We'll
> want to know (like Big Brother) a biography of the
> product and the ethics of the maker. We'll want to know
> the company's stand on the environment, how it regards
> animal testing, human rights, and other issues—rather
> than just a list of ingredients or a glimpse of an image.
> Listed prominently on the label, 800 numbers connecting
> the consumer to the corporation will be a way of life. (*The
> Popcorn Report* by Faith Popcorn. Doubleday 1991, p. 77)

Supporting Organic Growing

Organic growers are committed to ethical farming practices. According to many horticulturists and organic growers, the future of farming is learning how to grow native plants from seed, which is called *sustainable farming*. This approach to agriculture is centuries old. Sustainable farming creates a sustainable vegetation system or "web" that keeps rebuilding upon itself for decades. Planting in this way helps to renew and protect soil, allowing the diverse range of organisms—some even pests—to coexist within the food chain. When the food chain is left intact, parasites are taken care of by their natural predators, or natural repellents. Organic farmers therefore practice what's known as *companion planting*, which is simply ethical "biological pest management." In other words, if Vegetable A is always pestered by Beetle X, you simply plant Vegetable B next to it, which, together with Vegetable A, produces an odor that turns off Beetle X so that it doesn't go near either plant. Or, you can plant Weed A next to Vegetable A, which is a more tempting treat for Beetle X. Vegetable A grows beautifully, Weed A gets devoured, and then you simply hand-pick Weed A and throw it out at the end of the season. Companion planting is used to confuse insects, repel them or trap them. Companion planting is also used to make crops healthier. Vegetable A, for example, will grow better when it's beside Weed A, for reasons not completely understood.

But I don't want to be a farmer!
You don't have to be a farmer to eat organic produce. Hundreds of organic farmers, united under the Organic Growers Association or the Organic Trade Association, will be happy to sell you their organic produce, from vegetables and beef to clothing (made with cotton that was grown without pesticides). By buying organic spinach instead of spinach that was sprayed with endosulphan (a pesticide), you are supporting organic farming, eating well and saving the world—all at the same time. To find out where your organic farmers are, contact your local chapter of the Organic Growers Association or the Organic Trade Association listed in the resources section at the back of this book.

In your own backyard
While yes, you do have a beautiful flower garden that may be the envy of all your neighbors, but if you're using pesticides, you're part of the problem, not the solution, as they said in the 1960s. The Organic Growers and Organic Trade Associations have lots of literature available on organic insecticides and fungicides for lawns and gardens, as well as companion planting tips for the backyard (such as planting garlic beside roses).

Learning More about Bioengineered Food

Genetically altered produce and animals (where genes are manipulated for different growth results) are seen as one way to get around pesticides and diseases while improving food delivery. Scientists are concerned that by dicing and splicing various genes, ecological Frankensteins could be introduced into the environment, creating opportunities for exotic organisms and diseases to wreak havoc on our health. For example, in an effort to create strawberries that can grow in frost conditions, bioengineers unwittingly created a weed that can also grow in frost, which can interfere with other plants. Some scarier things have already been done, including cloning a sheep (Dolly); mixing sheep cells with goat cells; mixing pig cells with human cells; and mixing cattle, rat and human cells with carp, catfish, trout and salmon cells.

There is potential for bioengineered foods and genetic engineering to create very good things for the future: we may be able to clone extra organs, or perhaps find better treatments for cancer, or completely reinvent farming and do away with pesticides. But we ought to support this research in controlled laboratories. Right now, consumers are often unwitting and unwilling research participants in an ongoing experiment as we are buying altered fruits and vegetables that are not labeled as such.

The danger is in allowing these new breeds of plants or animals to breed or pollinate with their "original" species, spoiling the gene pools ever after. To find out whether your produce was genetically engineered, call the USDA information line at 202-720-2791 or Agriculture and Agrifood Canada at 613-952-8000.

What touches the earth touches the water and the food chain. But what touches our waters also touches the earth and the food chain—and our bodies. By learning about the state of our Great Lakes, we can use consumer power to clean them up so that maybe, one day, our *great* grandchildren can swim in them again.

The International Agency for Research on Cancer

Overall Evaluations of Carcinogenicity to Humans

The following lists are based on IARC research, which is considered the "gold standard" by which chemicals are evaluated in terms of carcinogenicity. This list is not intended for average people like you and me. So here's an explanation of what you're seeing. In square brackets are the chemical abstract numbers for each chemical (that's for scientists, not for us). In round brackets are the references to the relevant publication for each listing (this is a publication of all the studies done on that particular agent, chemical or group of agents), with a volume number, and year of publication (that's also for the scientists, and not for us). So, following the lists of Group 1, Group 2A and Group 2B is the complete list of references for your information, which can be accessed from the IARC's website at: *http://193.51.164.11/monoeval/allmonos.html*.

Group 1: Carcinogenic to humans (77)

Agents and groups of agents

Aflatoxins, naturally occurring [1402-68-2] (Vol. 56; 1993)
4-Aminobiphenyl [92-67-1] (Vol. 1, Suppl. 7; 1987)
Arsenic [7440-38-2] and arsenic compounds (Vol. 23, Suppl. 7; 1987)
(NB: This evaluation applies to the group of compounds as a whole and not necessarily to all individual compounds within the group)
Asbestos [1332-21-4] (Vol. 14, Suppl. 7; 1987)
Azathioprine [446-86-6] (Vol. 26, Suppl. 7; 1987)
Benzene [71-43-2] (Vol. 29, Suppl. 7; 1987)
Benzidine [92-87-5] (Vol. 29, Suppl. 7; 1987)
Beryllium [7440-41-7] and beryllium compounds (Vol. 58; 1993)
(NB: Evaluated as a group)
N,N-Bis(2-chloroethyl)-2-naphthylamine (Chlornaphazine) [494-03-1]
(Vol. 4, Suppl. 7; 1987)
Bis(chloromethyl)ether [542-88-1] and chloromethyl methyl ether [107-30-2] (technical-grade)
(Vol. 4, Suppl. 7; 1987)
1,4-Butanediol dimethanesulfonate (Busulphan; Myleran) [55-98-1] (Vol. 4, Suppl. 7; 1987)
Cadmium [7440-43-9] and cadmium compounds (Vol. 58; 1993)

(NB: Evaluated as a group)

Chlorambucil [305-03-3] (Vol. 26, Suppl. 7; 1987)

1-(2-Chloroethyl)-3-(4-methylcyclohexyl)-1-nitrosourea (Methyl-CCNU; Semustine) [13909-09-6] (Suppl. 7; 1987)

Chromium[VI] compounds (Vol. 49; 1990)

(NB: Evaluated as a group)

Ciclosporin [79217-60-0] (Vol. 50; 1990)

Cyclophosphamide [50-18-0] [6055-19-2] (Vol. 26, Suppl. 7; 1987)

Diethylstilboestrol [56-53-1] (Vol. 21, Suppl. 7; 1987)

Epstein-Barr virus (Vol. 70; 1997)

Erionite [66733-21-9] (Vol. 42, Suppl. 7; 1987)

Ethylene oxide [75-21-8] (Vol. 60; 1994)

(NB: Overall evaluation upgraded from 2A to 1 with supporting evidence from other data relevant to the evaluation of carcinogenicity and its mechanisms)

[Gamma Radiation: see X- and Gamma (g)-Radiation]

Helicobacter pylori (infection with) (Vol. 61; 1994)

Hepatitis B virus (chronic infection with) (Vol. 59; 1994)

Hepatitis C virus (chronic infection with) (Vol. 59; 1994)

Human immunodeficiency virus type 1 (infection with) (Vol. 67; 1996)

Human papillomavirus type 16 (Vol. 64; 1995)

Human papillomavirus type 18 (Vol. 64; 1995)

Human T-cell lymphotropic virus type I (Vol. 67; 1996)

Melphalan [148-82-3] (Vol. 9, Suppl. 7; 1987)

8-Methoxypsoralen (Methoxsalen) [298-81-7] plus ultraviolet A radiation (Vol. 24, Suppl. 7; 1987)

MOPP and other combined chemotherapy including alkylating agents (Suppl. 7; 1987)

Mustard gas (Sulfur mustard) [505-60-2] (Vol. 9, Suppl. 7; 1987)

2-Naphthylamine [91-59-8] (Vol. 4, Suppl. 7; 1987)

Neutrons (Vol. 75; 2000)

Nickel compounds (Vol. 49; 1990)

(NB: Evaluated as a group)

Oestrogen therapy, postmenopausal (Vol. 72; 1999)

Oestrogens, nonsteroidal (Suppl. 7; 1987)

(NB: This evaluation applies to the group of compounds as a whole and not necessarily to all individual compounds within the group)

Oestrogens, steroidal (Suppl. 7; 1987)

(NB: This evaluation applies to the group of compounds as a whole and

not necessarily to all individual compounds within the group)
Opisthorchis viverrini (infection with) (Vol. 61; 1994)
Oral contraceptives, combined (Vol. 72; 1999)
(NB: There is also conclusive evidence that these agents have a protective effect against cancers of the ovary and endometrium)
Oral contraceptives, sequential (Suppl. 7; 1987)
Radon [10043-92-2] and its decay products (Vol. 43; 1988)
Schistosoma haematobium (infection with) (Vol. 61; 1994)
Silica [14808-60-7], crystalline (inhaled in the form of quartz or cristo-balite from occupational sources) (Vol. 68; 1997)
Solar radiation (Vol. 55; 1992)
Talc containing asbestiform fibers (Vol. 42, Suppl. 7; 1987)
Tamoxifen [10540-29-1] (Vol. 66; 1996)
(NB: There is also conclusive evidence that this agent [tamoxifen] reduces the risk of contralateral breast cancer)
2,3,7,8-Tetrachlorodibenzo-*para*-dioxin [1746-01-6] (Vol. 69; 1997)
(NB: Overall evaluation upgraded from 2A to 1 with supporting evidence from other data relevant to the evaluation of carcinogenicity and its mechanisms)
Thiotepa [52-24-4] (Vol. 50; 1990)
Treosulfan [299-75-2] (Vol. 26, Suppl. 7; 1987)
Vinyl chloride [75-01-4] (Vol. 19, Suppl. 7; 1987)
X- and Gamma (g)-Radiation (Vol. 75; 2000)

Mixtures

Alcoholic beverages (Vol. 44; 1988)
Analgesic mixtures containing phenacetin (Suppl. 7; 1987)
Betel quid with tobacco (Vol. 37, Suppl. 7; 1987)
Coal-tar pitches [65996-93-2] (Vol. 35, Suppl. 7; 1987)
Coal-tars [8007-45-2] (Vol. 35, Suppl. 7; 1987)
Mineral oils, untreated and mildly treated (Vol. 33, Suppl. 7; 1987)
Salted fish (Chinese-style) (Vol. 56; 1993)
Shale-oils [68308-34-9] (Vol. 35, Suppl. 7; 1987)
Soots (Vol. 35, Suppl. 7; 1987)
Tobacco products, smokeless (Vol. 37, Suppl. 7; 1987)
Tobacco smoke (Vol. 38, Suppl. 7; 1987)
Wood dust (Vol. 62; 1995)

Exposure circumstances

Aluminium production (Vol. 34, Suppl. 7; 1987)

Auramine, manufacture of (Suppl. 7; 1987)

Boot and shoe manufacture and repair (Vol. 25, Suppl. 7; 1987)

Coal gasification (Vol. 34, Suppl. 7; 1987)

Coke production (Vol. 34, Suppl. 7; 1987)

Furniture and cabinet making (Vol. 25, Suppl. 7; 1987)

Haematite mining (underground) with exposure to radon (Vol. 1, Suppl. 7; 1987)

Iron and steel founding (Vol. 34, Suppl. 7; 1987)

Isopropanol manufacture (strong-acid process) (Suppl. 7; 1987)

Magenta, manufacture of (Vol. 57; 1993)

Painter (occupational exposure as a) (Vol. 47; 1989)

Rubber industry (Vol. 28, Suppl. 7; 1987)

Strong-inorganic-acid mists containing sulfuric acid (occupational exposure to) (Vol. 54; 1992)

Source: IARC. Posted to the Internet, April, 2000.

Group 2A: Probably carcinogenic to humans (59)

Agents and groups of agents

Acrylamide [79-06-1] (Vol. 60; 1994)
(NB: Overall evaluation upgraded from 2B to 2A with supporting evidence from other data relevant to the evaluation of carcinogenicity and its mechanisms)
Adriamycin [23214-92-8] (Vol. 10, Suppl. 7; 1987)
(NB: Overall evaluation upgraded from 2B to 2A with supporting evidence from other data relevant to the evaluation of carcinogenicity and its mechanisms)
Androgenic (anabolic) steroids (Suppl. 7; 1987)
Azacitidine [320-67-2] (Vol. 50; 1990)
(NB: Overall evaluation upgraded from 2B to 2A with supporting evidence from other data relevant to the evaluation of carcinogenicity and its mechanisms)
Benz[*a*]anthracene [56-55-3] (Vol. 32, Suppl. 7; 1987)
(NB: Overall evaluation upgraded from 2B to 2A with supporting evidence from other data relevant to the evaluation of carcinogenicity and its mechanisms)
Benzidine-based dyes (Suppl. 7; 1987)
(NB: Overall evaluation upgraded from 2B to 2A with supporting evidence from other data relevant to the evaluation of carcinogenicity and its mechanisms)
Benzo[*a*]pyrene [50-32-8] (Vol. 32, Suppl. 7; 1987)
(NB: Overall evaluation upgraded from 2B to 2A with supporting evidence from other data relevant to the evaluation of carcinogenicity and its mechanisms)
Bischloroethyl nitrosourea (BCNU) [154-93-8] (Vol. 26, Suppl. 7; 1987)
1,3-Butadiene [106-99-0] (Vol. 71; 1999)
Captafol [2425-06-1] (Vol. 53; 1991)
(NB: Overall evaluation upgraded from 2B to 2A with supporting evidence from other data relevant to the evaluation of carcinogenicity and its mechanisms)
Chloramphenicol [56-75-7] (Vol. 50; 1990)
(NB: Overall evaluation upgraded from 2B to 2A with supporting evidence from other data relevant to the evaluation of carcinogenicity and its mechanisms)
a-Chlorinated toluenes (benzal chloride [98-87-3], benzotrichloride [98-

07-7], benzyl chloride [100-44-7]) and benzoyl chloride [98-88-4] (combined exposures) (Vol. 29, Suppl. 7, Vol. 71; 1999)

1-(2-Chloroethyl)-3-cyclohexyl-1-nitrosourea (CCNU) [13010-47-4] (Vol. 26, Suppl. 7; 1987)

(NB: Overall evaluation upgraded from 2B to 2A with supporting evidence from other data relevant to the evaluation of carcinogenicity and its mechanisms)

para-Chloro-*ortho*-toluidine [95-69-2] and its strong acid salts (Vol. 48; 1990)

(NB: Evaluated as a group)

Chlorozotocin [54749-90-5] (Vol. 50; 1990)

(NB: Overall evaluation upgraded from 2B to 2A with supporting evidence from other data relevant to the evaluation of carcinogenicity and its mechanisms)

Cisplatin [15663-27-1] (Vol. 26, Suppl. 7; 1987)

(NB: Overall evaluation upgraded from 2B to 2A with supporting evidence from other data relevant to the evaluation of carcinogenicity and its mechanisms)

Clonorchis sinensis (infection with) (Vol. 61; 1994)

(NB: Overall evaluation upgraded from 2B to 2A with supporting evidence from other data relevant to the evaluation of carcinogenicity and its mechanisms)

Dibenz[a,h]anthracene [53-70-3] (Vol. 32, Suppl. 7; 1987)

(NB: Overall evaluation upgraded from 2B to 2A with supporting evidence from other data relevant to the evaluation of carcinogenicity and its mechanisms)

Diethyl sulfate [64-67-5] (Vol. 54, Vol. 71; 1999)

(NB: Overall evaluation upgraded from 2B to 2A with supporting evidence from other data relevant to the evaluation of carcinogenicity and its mechanisms)

Dimethylcarbamoyl chloride [79-44-7] (Vol. 12, Suppl. 7, Vol. 71; 1999)

(NB: Overall evaluation upgraded from 2B to 2A with supporting evidence from other data relevant to the evaluation of carcinogenicity and its mechanisms)

1,2-Dimethylhydrazine [540-73-8] (Vol. 4, Suppl. 7, Vol. 71; 1999)

(NB: Overall evaluation upgraded from 2B to 2A with supporting evidence from other data relevant to the evaluation of carcinogenicity and its mechanisms)

Dimethyl sulfate [77-78-1] (Vol. 4, Suppl. 7, Vol. 71; 1999)

(NB: Overall evaluation upgraded from 2B to 2A with supporting evidence from other data relevant to the evaluation of carcinogenicity and its mechanisms)

Epichlorohydrin [106-89-8] (Vol. 11, Suppl. 7, Vol. 71; 1999)

(NB: Overall evaluation upgraded from 2B to 2A with supporting evidence from other data relevant to the evaluation of carcinogenicity and its mechanisms)

Ethylene dibromide [106-93-4] (Vol. 15, Suppl. 7, Vol. 71; 1999)

(NB: Overall evaluation upgraded from 2B to 2A with supporting evidence from other data relevant to the evaluation of carcinogenicity and its mechanisms)

N-Ethyl-N-nitrosourea [759-73-9] (Vol. 17, Suppl. 7; 1987)

(NB: Overall evaluation upgraded from 2B to 2A with supporting evidence from other data relevant to the evaluation of carcinogenicity and its mechanisms)

Formaldehyde [50-00-0] (Vol. 62; 1995)

Human papillomavirus type 31 (Vol. 64; 1995)

Human papillomavirus type 33 (Vol. 64; 1995)

IQ (2-Amino-3-methylimidazo[4,5-f]quinoline) [76180-96-6] (Vol. 56; 1993)

(NB: Overall evaluation upgraded from 2B to 2A with supporting evidence from other data relevant to the evaluation of carcinogenicity and its mechanisms)

Kaposi's sarcoma herpes virus/human herpes virus 8 (Vol. 70; 1997)

5-Methoxypsoralen [484-20-8] (Vol. 40, Suppl. 7; 1987)

(NB: Overall evaluation upgraded from 2B to 2A with supporting evidence from other data relevant to the evaluation of carcinogenicity and its mechanisms)

4,4′-Methylene bis(2-chloroaniline) (MOCA) [101-14-4] (Vol. 57; 1993)

(NB: Overall evaluation upgraded from 2B to 2A with supporting evidence from other data relevant to the evaluation of carcinogenicity and its mechanisms)

Methyl methanesulfonate [66-27-3] (Vol. 7, Suppl. 7, Vol. 71; 1999)

(NB: Overall evaluation upgraded from 2B to 2A with supporting evidence from other data relevant to the evaluation of carcinogenicity and its mechanisms)

N-Methyl-N′-nitro-N-nitrosoguanidine (MNNG) [70-25-7] (Vol. 4, Suppl. 7; 1987)

(NB: Overall evaluation upgraded from 2B to 2A with supporting evidence from other data relevant to the evaluation of carcinogenicity and its mechanisms)

N-Methyl-N-nitrosourea [684-93-5] (Vol. 17, Suppl. 7; 1987)

(NB: Overall evaluation upgraded from 2B to 2A with supporting evidence from other data relevant to the evaluation of carcinogenicity and its mechanisms)

Nitrogen mustard [51-75-2] (Vol. 9, Suppl. 7; 1987)

N-Nitrosodiethylamine [55-18-5] (Vol. 17, Suppl. 7; 1987)

(NB: Overall evaluation upgraded from 2B to 2A with supporting evidence from other data relevant to the evaluation of carcinogenicity and its mechanisms)

N-Nitrosodimethylamine [62-75-9] (Vol. 17, Suppl. 7; 1987)

(NB: Overall evaluation upgraded from 2B to 2A with supporting evidence from other data relevant to the evaluation of carcinogenicity and its mechanisms)

Phenacetin [62-44-2] (Vol. 24, Suppl. 7; 1987)

Procarbazine hydrochloride [366-70-1] (Vol. 26, Suppl. 7; 1987)

(NB: Overall evaluation upgraded from 2B to 2A with supporting evidence from other data relevant to the evaluation of carcinogenicity and its mechanisms)

Styrene-7,8-oxide [96-09-3] (Vol. 60; 1994)

(NB: Overall evaluation upgraded from 2B to 2A with supporting evidence from other data relevant to the evaluation of carcinogenicity and its mechanisms)

Tetrachloroethylene [127-18-4] (Vol. 63; 1995)

Trichloroethylene [79-01-6] (Vol. 63; 1995)

1,2,3-Trichloropropane [96-18-4] (Vol. 63; 1995)

Tris(2,3-dibromopropyl) phosphate [126-72-7] (Vol. 20, Suppl. 7, Vol. 71; 1999)

(NB: Overall evaluation upgraded from 2B to 2A with supporting evidence from other data relevant to the evaluation of carcinogenicity and its mechanisms)

Ultraviolet radiation A (Vol. 55; 1992)

(NB: Overall evaluation upgraded from 2B to 2A with supporting evidence from other data relevant to the evaluation of carcinogenicity and its mechanisms)

Ultraviolet radiation B (Vol. 55; 1992)

(NB: Overall evaluation upgraded from 2B to 2A with supporting evidence from other data relevant to the evaluation of carcinogenicity and its mechanisms)

Ultraviolet radiation C (Vol. 55; 1992)

(NB: Overall evaluation upgraded from 2B to 2A with supporting evidence from other data relevant to the evaluation of carcinogenicity and its mechanisms)

Vinyl bromide [593-60-2] (Vol. 39, Suppl. 7, Vol. 71; 1999)

(NB: Overall evaluation upgraded from 2B to 2A with supporting evidence from other data relevant to the evaluation of carcinogenicity and its mechanisms)

Vinyl fluoride [75-02-5] (Vol. 63; 1995)

Mixtures

Creosotes [8001-58-9] (Vol. 35, Suppl. 7; 1987)

Diesel engine exhaust (Vol. 46; 1989)

Hot mate (Vol. 51; 1991)

Non-arsenical insecticides (occupational exposures in spraying and application of) (Vol. 53; 1991)

Polychlorinated biphenyls [1336-36-3] (Vol. 18, Suppl. 7; 1987)

Exposure circumstances

Art glass, glass containers and pressed ware (manufacture of) (Vol. 58; 1993)

Hairdresser or barber (occupational exposure as a) (Vol. 57; 1993)

Petroleum refining (occupational exposures in) (Vol. 45; 1989)

Sunlamps and sunbeds (use of) (Vol. 55; 1992)

Source: IARC. Posted to the Internet, April, 2000.

Group 2B: Possibly carcinogenic to humans (228)

Agents and groups of agents

A-a-C (2-Amino-9H-pyrido[2,3-b]indole) [26148-68-5] (Vol. 40, Suppl. 7; 1987)

Acetaldehyde [75-07-0] (Vol. 36, Suppl. 7, Vol. 71; 1999)

Acetamide [60-35-5] (Vol. 7, Suppl. 7, Vol. 71; 1999)

Acrylonitrile [107-13-1] (Vol. 71; 1999)

AF-2 [2-(2-Furyl)-3-(5-nitro-2-furyl)acrylamide] [3688-53-7] (Vol. 31, Suppl. 7; 1987)

Aflatoxin M1 [6795-23-9] (Vol. 56; 1993)

para-Aminoazobenzene [60-09-3] (Vol. 8, Suppl. 7; 1987)

ortho-Aminoazotoluene [97-56-3] (Vol. 8, Suppl. 7; 1987)

2-Amino-5-(5-nitro-2-furyl)-1,3,4-thiadiazole [712-68-5] (Vol. 7, Suppl. 7; 1987)

Amitrole [61-82-5] (Vol. 41, Suppl. 7; 1987)

ortho-Anisidine [90-04-0] (Vol. 73; 1999)

Antimony trioxide [1309-64-4] (Vol. 47; 1989)

Aramite® [140-57-8] (Vol. 5, Suppl. 7; 1987)

Auramine [492-80-8] (technical-grade) (Vol. 1, Suppl. 7; 1987)

Azaserine [115-02-6] (Vol. 10, Suppl. 7; 1987)

Aziridine [151-56-4] (Vol. 9, Suppl. 7, Vol. 71; 1999)

(NB: Overall evaluation upgraded from 3 to 2B with supporting evidence from other data relevant to the evaluation of carcinogenicity and its mechanisms)

Benzo[b]fluoranthene [205-99-2] (Vol. 32, Suppl. 7; 1987)

Benzo[j]fluoranthene [205-82-3] (Vol. 32, Suppl. 7; 1987)

Benzo[k]fluoranthene [207-08-9] (Vol. 32, Suppl. 7; 1987)

Benzofuran [271-89-6] (Vol. 63; 1995)

Benzyl violet 4B [1694-09-3] (Vol. 16, Suppl. 7; 1987)

Bleomycins [11056-06-7] (Vol. 26, Suppl. 7; 1987)

(NB: Overall evaluation upgraded from 3 to 2B with supporting evidence from other data relevant to the evaluation of carcinogenicity and its mechanisms)

Bracken fern (Vol. 40, Suppl. 7; 1987)

Bromodichloromethane [75-27-4] (Vol. 52, Vol. 71; 1999)

Butylated hydroxyanisole (BHA) [25013-16-5] (Vol. 40, Suppl. 7; 1987)

b-Butyrolactone [3068-88-0] (Vol. 11, Suppl. 7, Vol. 71; 1999)

Caffeic acid [331-39-5] (Vol. 56; 1993)

Carbon black [1333-86-4] (Vol. 65; 1996)
Carbon tetrachloride [56-23-5] (Vol. 20, Suppl. 7, Vol. 71; 1999)
Catechol [120-80-9] (Vol. 15, Suppl. 7, Vol. 71; 1999)
Ceramic fibers (Vol. 43; 1988)
Chlordane [57-74-9] (Vol. 53; 1991)
Chlordecone (Kepone) [143-50-0] (Vol. 20, Suppl. 7; 1987)
Chlorendic acid [115-28-6] (Vol. 48; 1990)
para-Chloroaniline [106-47-8] (Vol. 57; 1993)
Chloroform [67-66-3] (Vol. 73; 1999)
1-Chloro-2-methylpropene [513-37-1] (Vol. 63; 1995)
Chlorophenoxy herbicides (Vol. 41, Suppl. 7; 1987)
4-Chloro-ortho-phenylenediamine [95-83-0] (Vol. 27, Suppl. 7; 1987)
Chloroprene [126-99-8] (Vol. 71; 1999)
Chlorothalonil [1897-45-6] (Vol. 73; 1999)
CI Acid Red 114 [6459-94-5] (Vol. 57; 1993)
CI Basic Red 9 [569-61-9] (Vol. 57; 1993)
CI Direct Blue 15 [2429-74-5] (Vol. 57; 1993)
Citrus Red No. 2 [6358-53-8] (Vol. 8, Suppl. 7; 1987)
Cobalt [7440-48-4] and cobalt compounds (Vol. 52; 1991)
(NB: Evaluated as a group)
para-Cresidine [120-71-8] (Vol. 27, Suppl. 7; 1987)
Cycasin [14901-08-7] (Vol. 10, Suppl. 7; 1987)
Dacarbazine [4342-03-4] (Vol. 26, Suppl. 7; 1987)
Dantron (Chrysazin; 1,8-Dihydroxyanthraquinone) [117-10-2] (Vol. 50; 1990)
Daunomycin [20830-81-3] (Vol. 10, Suppl. 7; 1987)
DDT [p,p'-DDT, 50-29-3] (Vol. 53; 1991)
N,N'-Diacetylbenzidine [613-35-4] (Vol. 16, Suppl. 7; 1987)
2,4-Diaminoanisole [615-05-4] (Vol. 27, Suppl. 7; 1987)
4,4'-Diaminodiphenyl ether [101-80-4] (Vol. 29, Suppl. 7; 1987)
2,4-Diaminotoluene [95-80-7] (Vol. 16, Suppl. 7; 1987)
Dibenz[a,h]acridine [226-36-8] (Vol. 32, Suppl. 7; 1987)
Dibenz[a,j]acridine [224-42-0] (Vol. 32, Suppl. 7; 1987)
7H-Dibenzo[c,g]carbazole [194-59-2] (Vol. 32, Suppl. 7; 1987)
Dibenzo[a,e]pyrene [192-65-4] (Vol. 32, Suppl. 7; 1987)
Dibenzo[a,h]pyrene [189-64-0] (Vol. 32, Suppl. 7; 1987)
Dibenzo[a,i]pyrene [189-55-9] (Vol. 32, Suppl. 7; 1987)
Dibenzo[a,l]pyrene [191-30-0] (Vol. 32, Suppl. 7; 1987)
1,2-Dibromo-3-chloropropane [96-12-8] (Vol. 20, Suppl. 7, Vol. 71; 1999)

para-Dichlorobenzene [106-46-7] (Vol. 73; 1999)

(NB: Mechanistic data taken into account for making overall evaluation)

3,3'-Dichlorobenzidine [91-94-1] (Vol. 29, Suppl. 7; 1987)

3,3'-Dichloro-4,4'-diaminodiphenyl ether [28434-86-8] (Vol. 16, Suppl. 7; 1987)

1,2-Dichloroethane [107-06-2] (Vol. 20, Suppl. 7, Vol. 71; 1999)

Dichloromethane (methylene chloride) [75-09-2] (Vol. 71; 1999)

1,3-Dichloropropene [542-75-6] (technical-grade) (Vol. 41, Suppl. 7, Vol. 71; 1999)

Dichlorvos [62-73-7] (Vol. 53; 1991)

Di(2-ethylhexyl) phthalate [117-81-7] (Vol. 29, Suppl. 7; 1987)

1,2-Diethylhydrazine [1615-80-1] (Vol. 4, Suppl. 7, Vol. 71; 1999)

Diglycidyl resorcinol ether [101-90-6] (Vol. 36, Suppl. 7, Vol. 71; 1999)

Dihydrosafrole [94-58-6] (Vol. 10, Suppl. 7; 1987)

Diisopropyl sulfate [2973-10-6] (Vol. 54, Vol. 71; 1999)

3,3'-Dimethoxybenzidine (*ortho*-Dianisidine) [119-90-4] (Vol. 4, Suppl. 7; 1987)

para-Dimethylaminoazobenzene [60-11-7] (Vol. 8, Suppl. 7; 1987)

trans-2-[(Dimethylamino)methylimino]-5-[2-(5-nitro-2-furyl)-vinyl]-1,3,4-oxadiazole [25962-77-0]

(Vol. 7, Suppl. 7; 1987)

2,6-Dimethylaniline (2,6-Xylidine) [87-62-7] (Vol. 57; 1993)

3,3'-Dimethylbenzidine (*ortho*-Tolidine) [119-93-7] (Vol. 1, Suppl. 7; 1987)

1,1-Dimethylhydrazine [57-14-7] (Vol. 4, Suppl. 7, Vol. 71; 1999)

3,7-Dinitrofluoranthene [105735-71-5] (Vol. 65; 1996)

3,9-Dinitrofluoranthene [22506-53-2] (Vol. 65; 1996)

1,6-Dinitropyrene [42397-64-8] (Vol. 46; 1989)

1,8-Dinitropyrene [42397-65-9] (Vol. 46; 1989)

2,4-Dinitrotoluene [121-14-2] (Vol. 65; 1996)

2,6-Dinitrotoluene [606-20-2] (Vol. 65; 1996)

1,4-Dioxane [123-91-1] (Vol. 11, Suppl. 7, Vol. 71; 1999)

Disperse Blue 1 [2475-45-8] (Vol. 48; 1990)

1,2-Epoxybutane [106-88-7] (Vol. 47, Vol. 71; 1999)

(NB: Overall evaluation upgraded from 3 to 2B with supporting evidence from other data relevant to the evaluation of carcinogenicity and its mechanisms)

Ethyl acrylate [140-88-5] (Vol. 39, Suppl. 7, Vol. 71; 1999)

Ethylene thiourea [96-45-7] (Vol. 7, Suppl. 7; 1987)

Ethyl methanesulfonate [62-50-0] (Vol. 7, Suppl. 7; 1987)

Foreign bodies, implanted in tissues (Vol. 74; 1999)

Polymeric, prepared as thin smooth films (with the exception of poly[glycolic acid])

Metallic, prepared as thin smooth films

Metallic cobalt, metallic nickel and an alloy powder containing 66-67% nickel, 13-16% chromium and 7% iron

2-(2-Formylhydrazino)-4-(5-nitro-2-furyl)thiazole [3570-75-0] (Vol. 7, Suppl. 7; 1987)

Furan [110-00-9] (Vol. 63; 1995)

Glasswool (Vol. 43; 1988)

Glu-P-1 (2-Amino-6-methyldipyrido[1,2-*a*:3',2'-*d*]imidazole) [67730-11-4] (Vol. 40, Suppl. 7; 1987)

Glu-P-2 (2-Aminodipyrido[1,2-*a*:3',2'-*d*]imidazole) [67730-10-3] (Vol. 40, Suppl. 7; 1987)

Glycidaldehyde [765-34-4] (Vol. 11, Suppl. 7, Vol. 71; 1999)

Griseofulvin [126-07-8] (Vol. 10, Suppl. 7; 1987)

HC Blue No. 1 [2784-94-3] (Vol. 57; 1993)

Heptachlor [76-44-8] (Vol. 53; 1991)

Hexachlorobenzene [118-74-1] (Vol. 20, Suppl. 7; 1987)

Hexachloroethane [67-72-1] (Vol. 73; 1999)

Hexachlorocyclohexanes (Vol. 20, Suppl. 7; 1987)

Hexamethylphosphoramide [680-31-9] (Vol. 15, Suppl. 7, Vol. 71; 1999)

Human immunodeficiency virus type 2 (infection with) (Vol. 67; 1996)

Human papillomaviruses: some types other than 16, 18, 31 and 33 (Vol. 64; 1995)

Hydrazine [302-01-2] (Vol. 4, Suppl. 7, Vol. 71; 1999)

Indeno[1,2,3-*cd*]pyrene [193-39-5] (Vol. 32, Suppl. 7; 1987)

Iron-dextran complex [9004-66-4] (Vol. 2, Suppl. 7; 1987)

Isoprene [78-79-5] (Vol. 60, Vol. 71; 1999)

Lasiocarpine [303-34-4] (Vol. 10, Suppl. 7; 1987)

Lead [7439-92-1] and lead compounds, inorganic (Vol. 23, Suppl. 7; 1987)

(NB: Evaluated as a group)

Magenta [632-99-5] (containing CI Basic Red 9) (Vol. 57; 1993)

MeA-*a*-C (2-Amino-3-methyl-9*H*-pyrido[2,3-*b*]indole) [68006-83-7] (Vol. 40, Suppl. 7; 1987)

Medroxyprogesterone acetate [71-58-9] (Vol. 21, Suppl. 7; 1987)

MeIQ (2-Amino-3,4-dimethylimidazo[4,5-*f*]quinoline) [77094-11-2] (Vol.

56; 1993)

MeIQx (2-Amino-3,8-dimethylimidazo[4,5-f]quinoxaline) [77500-04-0] (Vol. 56; 1993)

Merphalan [531-76-0] (Vol. 9, Suppl. 7; 1987)

2-Methylaziridine (Propyleneimine) [75-55-8] (Vol. 9, Suppl. 7, Vol. 71; 1999)

Methylazoxymethanol acetate [592-62-1] (Vol. 10, Suppl. 7; 1987)

5-Methylchrysene [3697-24-3] (Vol. 32, Suppl. 7; 1987)

4,4'-Methylene bis(2-methylaniline) [838-88-0] (Vol. 4, Suppl. 7; 1987)

4,4'-Methylenedianiline [101-77-9] (Vol. 39, Suppl. 7; 1987)

Methylmercury compounds (Vol. 58; 1993)

(NB: Evaluated as a group)

2-Methyl-1-nitroanthraquinone [129-15-7] (uncertain purity) (Vol. 27, Suppl. 7; 1987)

N-Methyl-N-nitrosourethane [615-53-2] (Vol. 4, Suppl. 7; 1987)

Methylthiouracil [56-04-2] (Vol. 7, Suppl. 7; 1987)

Metronidazole [443-48-1] (Vol. 13, Suppl. 7; 1987)

Mirex [2385-85-5] (Vol. 20, Suppl. 7; 1987)

Mitomycin C [50-07-7] (Vol. 10, Suppl. 7; 1987)

Monocrotaline [315-22-0] (Vol. 10, Suppl. 7; 1987)

5-(Morpholinomethyl)-3-[(5-nitrofurfurylidene)amino]-2-oxazolidinone [3795-88-8] (Vol. 7, Suppl. 7; 1987)

Nafenopin [3771-19-5] (Vol. 24, Suppl. 7; 1987)

Nickel, metallic [7440-02-0] and alloys (Vol. 49; 1990)

Niridazole [61-57-4] (Vol. 13, Suppl. 7; 1987)

Nitrilotriacetic acid [139-13-9] and its salts (Vol. 73; 1999)

(NB: Evaluated as a group)

5-Nitroacenaphthene [602-87-9] (Vol. 16, Suppl. 7; 1987)

2-Nitroanisole [91-23-6] (Vol. 65; 1996)

Nitrobenzene [98-95-3] (Vol. 65; 1996)

6-Nitrochrysene [7496-02-8] (Vol. 46; 1989)

Nitrofen [1836-75-5] (technical-grade) (Vol. 30, Suppl. 7; 1987)

2-Nitrofluorene [607-57-8] (Vol. 46; 1989)

1-[(5-Nitrofurfurylidene)amino]-2-imidazolidinone [555-84-0] (Vol. 7, Suppl. 7; 1987)

N-[4-(5-Nitro-2-furyl)-2-thiazolyl]acetamide [531-82-8] (Vol. 7, Suppl. 7; 1987)

Nitrogen mustard N-oxide [126-85-2] (Vol. 9, Suppl. 7; 1987)

2-Nitropropane [79-46-9] (Vol. 29, Suppl. 7, Vol. 71; 1999)

1-Nitropyrene [5522-43-0] (Vol. 46; 1989)

4-Nitropyrene [57835-92-4] (Vol. 46; 1989)

N-Nitrosodi-n-butylamine [924-16-3] (Vol. 17, Suppl. 7; 1987)

N-Nitrosodiethanolamine [1116-54-7] (Vol. 17, Suppl. 7; 1987)

N-Nitrosodi-n-propylamine [621-64-7] (Vol. 17, Suppl. 7; 1987)

3-(N-Nitrosomethylamino)propionitrile [60153-49-3] (Vol. 37, Suppl. 7; 1987)

4-(N-Nitrosomethylamino)-1-(3-pyridyl)-1-butanone (NNK) [64091-91-4] (Vol. 37, Suppl. 7; 1987)

N-Nitrosomethylethylamine [10595-95-6] (Vol. 17, Suppl. 7; 1987)

N-Nitrosomethylvinylamine [4549-40-0] (Vol. 17, Suppl. 7; 1987)

N-Nitrosomorpholine [59-89-2] (Vol. 17, Suppl. 7; 1987)

N'-Nitrosonornicotine [16543-55-8] (Vol. 37, Suppl. 7; 1987)

N-Nitrosopiperidine [100-75-4] (Vol. 17, Suppl. 7; 1987)

N-Nitrosopyrrolidine [930-55-2] (Vol. 17, Suppl. 7; 1987)

N-Nitrososarcosine [13256-22-9] (Vol. 17, Suppl. 7; 1987)

Ochratoxin A [303-47-9] (Vol. 56; 1993)

Oestrogen-progestogen therapy, postmenopausal (Vol. 72; 1999)

Oil Orange SS [2646-17-5] (Vol. 8, Suppl. 7; 1987)

Oxazepam [604-75-1] (Vol. 66; 1996)

Palygorskite (attapulgite) [12174-11-7] (long fibers, > 5 micrometers) (Vol. 68; 1997)

Panfuran S [794-93-4] (containing dihydroxymethylfuratrizine) (Vol. 24, Suppl. 7; 1987)

Phenazopyridine hydrochloride [136-40-3] (Vol. 24, Suppl. 7; 1987)

Phenobarbital [50-06-6] (Vol. 13, Suppl. 7; 1987)

Phenoxybenzamine hydrochloride [63-92-3] (Vol. 24, Suppl. 7; 1987)

Phenyl glycidyl ether [122-60-1] (Vol. 47, Vol. 71; 1999)

Phenytoin [57-41-0] (Vol. 66; 1996)

PhIP (2-Amino-1-methyl-6-phenylimidazo[4,5-b]pyridine) [105650-23-5] (Vol. 56; 1993)

Polychlorophenols and their sodium salts (mixed exposures) (Vol. 41, Suppl. 7, Vol. 53, Vol. 71; 1999)

Ponceau MX [3761-53-3] (Vol. 8, Suppl. 7; 1987)

Ponceau 3R [3564-09-8] (Vol. 8, Suppl. 7; 1987)

Potassium bromate [7758-01-2] (Vol. 73; 1999)

Progestins (Suppl. 7; 1987)

Progestogen-only contraceptives (Vol. 72; 1999)

1,3-Propane sultone [1120-71-4] (Vol. 4, Suppl. 7, Vol. 71; 1999) b-Propiolactone [57-57-8] (Vol. 4, Suppl. 7, Vol. 71; 1999)

Propylene oxide [75-56-9] (Vol. 60; 1994)

Propylthiouracil [51-52-5] (Vol. 7, Suppl. 7; 1987)

Rockwool (Vol. 43; 1988)

Safrole [94-59-7] (Vol. 10, Suppl. 7; 1987)

Schistosoma japonicum (infection with) (Vol. 61; 1994)

Slagwool (Vol. 43; 1988)

Sodium *ortho*-phenylphenate [132-27-4] (Vol. 73; 1999)

Sterigmatocystin [10048-13-2] (Vol. 10, Suppl. 7; 1987)

Streptozotocin [18883-66-4] (Vol. 17, Suppl. 7; 1987)

Styrene [100-42-5] (Vol. 60; 1994)

(NB: Overall evaluation upgraded from 3 to 2B with supporting evidence from other data relevant to the evaluation of carcinogenicity and its mechanisms)

Sulfallate [95-06-7] (Vol. 30, Suppl. 7; 1987)

Tetrafluoroethylene [116-14-3] (Vol. 19, Suppl. 7, Vol. 71; 1999)

Tetranitromethane [509-14-8] (Vol. 65; 1996)

Thioacetamide [62-55-5] (Vol. 7, Suppl. 7; 1987)

4,4'-Thiodianiline [139-65-1] (Vol. 27, Suppl. 7; 1987)

Thiourea [62-56-6] (Vol. 7, Suppl. 7; 1987)

Toluene diisocyanates [26471-62-5] (Vol. 39, Suppl. 7, Vol. 71; 1999)

ortho-Toluidine [95-53-4] (Vol. 27, Suppl. 7; 1987)

Toxins derived from *Fusarium moniliforme* (Vol. 56; 1993)

Trichlormethine (Trimustine hydrochloride) [817-09-4] (Vol. 50; 1990)

Trp-P-1 (3-Amino-1,4-dimethyl-5*H*-pyrido[4,3-*b*]indole) [62450-06-0] (Vol. 31, Suppl. 7; 1987)

Trp-P-2 (3-Amino-1-methyl-5*H*-pyrido[4,3-*b*]indole) [62450-07-1] (Vol. 31, Suppl. 7; 1987)

Trypan blue [72-57-1] (Vol. 8, Suppl. 7; 1987)

Uracil mustard [66-75-1] (Vol. 9, Suppl. 7; 1987)

Urethane [51-79-6] (Vol. 7, Suppl. 7; 1987)

Vinyl acetate [108-05-4] (Vol. 63; 1995)

4-Vinylcyclohexene [100-40-3] (Vol. 60; 1994)

4-Vinylcyclohexene diepoxide [106-87-6] (Vol. 60; 1994)

Mixtures

Bitumens [8052-42-4], extracts of steam-refined and air-refined (Vol. 35, Suppl. 7; 1987)

Carrageenan [9000-07-1], degraded (Vol. 31, Suppl. 7; 1987)

Chlorinated paraffins of average carbon chain length C12 and average degree of chlorination approximately 60% (Vol. 48; 1990)

Coffee (urinary bladder) (Vol. 51; 1991)

(NB: There is some evidence of an inverse relationship between coffee drinking and cancer of the large bowel; coffee drinking could not be classified as to its carcinogenicity to other organs)

Diesel fuel, marine (Vol. 45; 1989)

(NB: Overall evaluation upgraded from 3 to 2B with supporting evidence from other data relevant to the evaluation of carcinogenicity and its mechanisms)

Engine exhaust, gasoline (Vol. 46; 1989)

Fuel oils, residual (heavy) (Vol. 45; 1989)

Gasoline (Vol. 45; 1989)

(NB: Overall evaluation upgraded from 3 to 2B with supporting evidence from other data relevant to the evaluation of carcinogenicity and its mechanisms)

Pickled vegetables (traditional in Asia) (Vol. 56; 1993)

Polybrominated biphenyls [Firemaster BP-6, 59536-65-1] (Vol. 41, Suppl. 7; 1987)

Toxaphene (Polychlorinated camphenes) [8001-35-2] (Vol. 20, Suppl. 7; 1987)

Welding fumes (Vol. 49; 1990)

Exposure circumstances

Carpentry and joinery (Vol. 25, Suppl. 7; 1987)

Dry cleaning (occupational exposures in) (Vol. 63; 1995)

Printing processes (occupational exposures in) (Vol. 65; 1996)

Textile manufacturing industry (work in) (Vol. 48; 1990)

Source: IARC. Posted to the Internet, April, 2000.

IARC Monographs
on the Evaluation of Carcinogenic Risks
to Humans and their Supplements:
A complete list

Monographs

Volume 1
Some Inorganic Substances, Chlorinated Hydrocarbons, Aromatic Amines,
N-Nitroso Compounds, and Natural Products

1972; 184 pages
ISBN 92 832 1201 0 (out of print)

Volume 2
Some Inorganic and Organometallic Compounds

1973; 181 pages
ISBN 92 832 1202 9 (out of print)

Volume 3
Certain Polycyclic Aromatic Hydrocarbons and Heterocyclic Compounds

1973; 271 pages
ISBN 92 832 1203 7 (out of print)

Volume 4
Some Aromatic Amines, Hydrazine and Related Substances, N-Nitroso
Compounds and Miscellaneous Alkylating Agents

1974; 286 pages
ISBN 92 832 1204 5
US$ 21

Volume 5
Some Organochlorine Pesticides

1974; 241 pages
ISBN 92 832 1205 3 (out of print)

Volume 6
Sex Hormones

1974; 243 pages
ISBN 92 832 1206 1 (out of print)

US$ 16

Volume 7
Some Anti-Thyroid and Related Substances, Nitrofurans and Industrial Chemicals

1974; 326 pages
ISBN 92 832 1207 X (out of print)
US$ 28

Volume 8
Some Aromatic Azo Compounds

1975; 357 pages
ISBN 92 832 1208 8
US$ 38

Volume 9
Some Aziridines, N-, S- and O-Mustards and Selenium

1975; 268 pages
ISBN 92 832 1209 6
US$ 28

Volume 10
Some Naturally Occurring Substances

1976; 353 pages
ISBN 92 832 1210 X (out of print)

Volume 11
Cadmium, Nickel, Some Epoxides, Miscellaneous Industrial Chemicals and General Considerations on Volatile Anaesthetics

1976; 306 pages
ISBN 92 832 1211 8 (out of print)

Volume 12
Some Carbamates, Thiocarbamates and Carbazides

1976; 282 pages
ISBN 92 832 1212 6
US$ 35

Volume 13
Some Miscellaneous Pharmaceutical Substances

1977; 255 pages

ISBN 92 832 1213 4
US$ 31

Volume 14
Asbestos

1977; 106 pages
ISBN 92 832 1214 2 (out of print)

Volume 15
Some Fumigants, the Herbicides 2,4-D and 2,4,5-T, Chlorinated
Dibenzodioxins and Miscellaneous Industrial Chemicals

1977; 354 pages
ISBN 92 832 1215 0 (out of print)
US$ 72

Volume 16
Some Aromatic Amines and Related Nitro Compounds - Hair Dyes,
Coloring Agents and Miscellaneous Industrial Chemicals

1978; 400 pages
ISBN 92 832 1216 9
US$ 52

Volume 17
Some N-Nitroso Compounds

1978; 365 pages
ISBN 92 832 1217 7
US$ 52

Volume 18
Polychlorinated Biphenyls and Polybrominated Biphenyls

1978; 140 pages
ISBN 92 832 1218 5
US$ 21

Volume 19
Some Monomers, Plastics and Synthetic Elastomers, and Acrolein

1979; 513 pages
ISBN 92 832 1219 3 (out of print)

Volume 20

Some Halogenated Hydrocarbons

1979; 609 pages
ISBN 92 832 1220 7 (out of print)

Volume 21
Sex Hormones (II)

1979; 583 pages
ISBN 92 832 1521 4
US$ 62

Volume 22
Some Non-Nutritive Sweetening Agents

1980; 208 pages
ISBN 92 832 1522 2
US$ 26

Volume 23
Some Metals and Metallic Compounds

1980; 438 pages
ISBN 92 832 1523 0 (out of print)
US$ 43

Volume 24
Some Pharmaceutical Drugs

1980; 337 pages
ISBN 92 832 1524 9
US$ 41

Volume 25
Wood, Leather and Some Associated Industries

1981; 412 pages
ISBN 92 832 1525 7
US$ 62

Volume 26
Some Antineoplastic and Immunosuppressive Agents

1981; 411 pages
ISBN 92 832 1526 5
US$ 65

Volume 27

Some Aromatic Amines, Anthraquinones and Nitroso Compounds, and
Inorganic Fluorides Used in Drinking Water and Dental Preparations

1982; 341 pages
ISBN 92 832 1527 3
US$ 41

Volume 28
The Rubber Industry

1982; 486 pages
ISBN 92 832 1528 1
US$ 72

Volume 29
Some Industrial Chemicals and Dyestuffs

1982; 416 pages
ISBN 92 832 1529 X
US$ 62

Volume 30
Miscellaneous Pesticides

1983; 424 pages
ISBN 92 832 1530 3
US$ 62

Volume 31
Some Food Additives, Feed Additives and Naturally Occurring Substances

1983; 314 pages
ISBN 92 832 1531 1
US$ 57

Volume 32
Polynuclear Aromatic Compounds, Part 1: Chemical, Environmental and
Experimental Data

1983; 477 pages
ISBN 92 832 1532 X
US$ 57

Volume 33
Polynuclear Aromatic Compounds, Part 2: Carbon Blacks, Mineral Oils

(Lubricant Base Oils and Derived Products) and Some Nitroarenes

1984; 245 pages
ISBN 92 832 1533 8 (out of print)
US$ 22

Volume 34
Polynuclear Aromatic Compounds, Part 3: Industrial Exposures in Aluminium Production, Coal Gasification, Coke Production, and Iron and Steel Founding

1984; 219 pages
ISBN 92 832 1534 6
US$ 41

Volume 35
Polynuclear Aromatic Compounds, Part 4: Bitumens, Coal-Tars and Derived Products, Shale-Oils and Soots

1985; 271 pages
ISBN 92 832 1535 4
US$ 60

Volume 36
Allyl Compounds, Aldehydes, Epoxides and Peroxides

1985; 369 pages
ISBN 92 832 1536 2
US$ 66

Volume 37
Tobacco Habits Other than Smoking; Betel-Quid and Areca-Nut Chewing; and Some Related Nitrosamines

1985; 291 pages
ISBN 92 832 1537 0
US$ 66

Volume 38
Tobacco Smoking

1986; 421 pages
ISBN 92 832 1538 9
US$ 72

Volume 39
Some Chemicals Used in Plastics and Elastomers

1986; 403 pages
ISBN 92 832 1239 8
US$ 72

Volume 40
Some Naturally Occurring and Synthetic Food Components,
Furocoumarins and Ultraviolet Radiation

1986; 444 pages
ISBN 92 832 1240 1
US$ 72

Volume 41
Some Halogenated Hydrocarbons and Pesticide Exposures

1986; 434 pages
ISBN 92 832 1241 X
US$ 72

Volume 42
Silica and Some Silicates

1987; 289 pages
ISBN 92 832 1242 8
US$ 62

Volume 43
Man-Made Mineral Fibers and Radon

1988; 300 pages
ISBN 92 832 1243 6
US$ 62

Volume 44
Alcohol Drinking

1988; 416 pages
ISBN 92 832 1244 4
US$ 72

Volume 45
Occupational Exposures in Petroleum Refining; Crude Oil and Major
Petroleum Fuels

1989; 322 pages
ISBN 92 832 1245 2
US$ 62

Volume 46
Diesel and Gasoline Engine Exhausts and Some Nitroarenes

1989; 458 pages
ISBN 92 832 1246 0
US$ 72

Volume 47
Some Organic Solvents, Resin Monomers and Related Compounds,
Pigments and Occupational Exposures in Paint Manufacture and Painting

1989; 535 pages
ISBN 92 832 1247 9
US$ 81

Volume 48
Some Flame Retardants and Textile Chemicals,
and Exposures in the Textile Manufacturing Industry

1990; 345 pages
ISBN 92 832 1248 7
US$ 62

Volume 49
Chromium, Nickel and Welding

1990; 677 pages
ISBN 92 832 1249 5
US$ 91

Volume 50
Some Pharmaceutical Drugs

1990; 415 pages
ISBN 92 832 1259 9
US$ 72

Volume 51
Coffee, Tea, Mate, Methylxanthines and Methylglyoxal

1991; 513 pages
ISBN 92 832 1251 7

US$ 76

Volume 52
Chlorinated Drinking-water; Chlorination By-products; Some Other
Halogenated Compounds; Cobalt and Cobalt Compounds

1991; 544 pages
ISBN 92 832 1252 5
US$ 76

Volume 53
Occupational Exposures in Insecticide Application, and Some Pesticides

1991; 612 pages
ISBN 92 832 1253 3
US$ 91

Volume 54
Occupational Exposures to Mists and Vapors from Strong Inorganic Acids;
and Other Industrial Chemicals

1992; 336 pages
ISBN 92 832 1254 1
US$ 62

Volume 55
Solar and Ultraviolet Radiation

1992; 316 pages
ISBN 92 832 1255 X
US$ 62

Volume 56
Some Naturally Occurring Substances: Food Items and Constituents,
Heterocyclic Aromatic Amines and Mycotoxins

1993; 599 pages
ISBN 92 832 1256 8
US$ 82

Volume 57
Occupational Exposures of Hairdressers and Barbers and Personal Use of
Hair Colorants; Some Hair Dyes, Cosmetic Colorants, Industrial Dyestuffs
and Aromatic Amines

1993; 427 pages

ISBN 92 832 1257 6
US$ 65

Volume 58
Beryllium, Cadmium, Mercury, and Exposures in the Glass Manufacturing
Industry

1994; 444 pages
ISBN 92 832 1258 4
US$ 65

Volume 59
Hepatitis Viruses

1994; 286 pages
ISBN 92 832 1259 2
US$ 56

Volume 60
Some Industrial Chemicals

1994; 560 pages
ISBN 92 832 1260 6
US$ 78

Volume 61
Schistosomes, Liver Flukes and *Helicobacter pylori*

1994; 280 pages
ISBN 92 832 1261 4
US$ 60

Volume 62
Wood dust and Formaldehyde

1995; 405 pages
ISBN 92 832 1262 2
US$ 69

Volume 63
Dry cleaning, Some Chlorinated Solvents and Other Industrial Chemicals

1995; 558 pages
ISBN 92 832 1263 0
US$ 78

Volume 64

Human Papillomaviruses

1995; 409 pages
ISBN 92 832 1264 9
US$ 69

Volume 65
Printing Processes and Printing Inks, Carbon Black and Some Nitrocompounds

1996; 578 pages
ISBN 92 832 1265 7
US$ 78

Volume 66
Some Pharmaceutical Drugs

1996; 514 pages
ISBN 92 832 1266 5
US$ 69

Volume 67
Human Immunodeficiency Viruses and Human T-Cell Lymphotropic Viruses

1996; 424 pages
ISBN 92 832 1267 3
US$ 69

Volume 68
Silica, Some Silicates, Coal Dust and *para*-Aramid Fibrils

1997; 506 pages
ISBN 92 832 1268 1
US$ 69

Volume 69
Polychlorinated Dibenzo-*para*-Dioxins and Polychlorinated Dibenzofurans

1997; 666 pages
ISBN 92 832 1269 X
US$ 69

Volume 70
Epstein-Barr Virus and Kaposi's Sarcoma Herpesvirus/Human Herpesvirus

8

1997; 524 pages
ISBN 92 832 1270 3
US$ 69

Volume 71
Re-evaluation of Some Organic Chemicals, Hydrazine and Hydrogen
Peroxide

1999; 1589 pages
ISBN 92 832 1271 1

Volume 72
Hormonal Contraception and Post-menopausal Hormonal Therapy
1999; 660 pages
ISBN 92 832 1272 X

Volume 73
Some Chemicals that Cause Tumors of the Kidney or Urinary Bladder in
Rodents, and Some Other Substances

1999; 674 pages
ISBN 92 832 1273 8

Volume 74
Surgical Implants and Other Foreign Bodies

1999; 409 pages
ISBN 92 832 1274 6

Volume 75
Ionizing Radiation, Part 1: X- and Gamma (g)-Radiation, and Neutrons

2000; 492 pages
ISBN 92 832 1275 4

Supplements to the Monographs

Supplement No. 1
Chemicals and Industrial Processes Associated with Cancer in Humans
(IARC Monographs, Volumes 1 to 20)

1979; 71 pages
ISBN 92 832 1404 8 (out of print)

US$ 6

Supplement No. 2
Long-Term and Short-Term Screening Assays for Carcinogens: A Critical
Appraisal

1980; 426 pages
ISBN 92 832 1404 8
US$ 34

Supplement No. 3
Cross Index of Synonyms and Trade Names in Volumes 1 to 26

1982; 199 pages
ISBN 92 832 1405 6 (out of print)
US$ 29

Supplement No. 4
Chemicals, Industrial Processes and Industries Associated with Cancer in
Humans (IARC Monographs, Volumes 1 to 29)

1982; 292 pages
ISBN 92 832 1407 2 (out of print)
US$ 29

Supplement No. 5
Cross Index of Synonyms and Trade Names in Volumes 1 to 36

1985; 259 pages
ISBN 92 832 1408 0 (out of print)
US$ 20

Supplement No. 6
Genetic and Related Effects: An Updating of Selected IARC Monographs
from Volumes 1 to 42

1987; 729 pages
ISBN 92 832 1409 9
US$ 76

Supplement No. 7
Overall Evaluations of Carcinogenicity: An Updating of IARC Monographs
Volumes 1 to 42

1987; 440 pages
ISBN 92 832 1411 0

Stopping Cancer at the Source

US$ 62

Supplement No. 8
Cross Index of Synonyms and Trade Names in Volumes 1 to 46

1989; 346 pages
ISBN 92 832 1417 X
US$ 57

9
GREAT LAKES, BIG MESS

The Great Lakes Basin is home to some 36 million people, and is the largest body of freshwater on earth. If you're living in Ontario or any of the eight Great Lakes U.S. states (Minnesota, Wisconsin, Michigan, Illinois, Indiana, Ohio, New York and Pennsylvania), your health is at risk due to the presence of several hundred contaminants in the Great Lakes Basin, a dozen of which have been identified as really serious, such as PCBs and dioxins. The contaminant levels in the breast milk of Canadian women living in this region show that for suckling infants, daily intake of PCBs and dioxins (or dioxin-like contaminants) may exceed established guidelines for human exposure. But the alternative to breastfeeding—formula feeding—has even more serious health consequences for babies. More babies will die from digestive problems associated with formula than from the contaminants they're exposed to through breastfeeding, so health promotion experts still recommend breastfeeding to women living in these regions.

Another health paradox looms in the Great Lakes Basin: eating fish from the Great Lakes is a major source of carcinogens in local residents because these toxins bioaccumulate in the fish. But, for so many of us, heart-smart diets depend on consuming fish oils from fatty fish—the very fish that swim in the Great Lakes. We need their fat to protect us from heart disease, so we must weigh the risks of contamination against the risk of heart disease. There are no easy answers other than trying to clean up the mess.

What are the health consequences of Great Lakes toxins? In terms of cancer, we are looking at higher incidences of breast, testicular and prostate cancers due to the estrogenic toxins (i.e., toxins that break down into an estrogenic mimic) that are rampant in Great Lakes waters. Other cancers, such as bladder, thyroid and colon, are also elevated in these regions. There are higher risks of infertility in this population. Women are more likely to develop endometriosis and fibroids, which thrive on estrogen. This was shown in a recent study surveying 575 couples trying to conceive who regularly ate fish from heavily polluted Lake Ontario. These couples were 25 percent less likely to conceive each month. New York State has been advising women of childbearing age to avoid Lake Ontario fish for some time. Lake Ontario is known for its high concentrations of PCBs and other compounds, which can have hormone-like effects that disrupt a woman's fertility. Researchers form the State University of New York at Buffalo published the findings of this study in the July, 2000 issue of *Epidemiology*.

Meanwhile, Great Lakes baby boys are more likely to be born with undescended testicles, and then, as adults, could even be infertile due to low sperm counts. Fetuses exposed to these toxins are at greater risk for developmental disabilities. We also have too much harmful bacteria floating around, which come from the sewage pumped into these waters over the years. These are public health hazards, too.

This chapter is based on the recommendations of the Eighth Biennial Report on Great Lakes Water Quality, Under the Great Lakes Water Quality Agreement of 1978 to the Governments of the United States and Canada and the State and Provincial Governments of the Great Lakes Basin, released by the International Joint Commission in 1996. It also includes information from a unique 1998 report entitled: A State of Knowledge Report on the Effects of Human Health in the Great Lakes Basin, published by Health Canada in cooperation with the Great Lakes Health Effects Program, Environmental Health Effects Division of Health Canada.

A BRIEF HISTORY OF GREAT LAKES WATER QUALITY

Just in case you're not a geography whiz, the Great Lakes comprise: Lake Ontario (the source of the St. Lawrence River), Lake Erie, Lake Huron, Lake Michigan and Lake Superior. These waters and the lands that drain into these waters form what's known as the Great Lakes Basin, and when discussing environmental concerns, the term "Great Lakes Basin Ecosystem" is used. This is a huge territory that consists of area in eight U.S. states and Ontario, plus Quebec, which is connected to the basin through the St. Lawrence River. A number of large industrial cities lie along the Great Lakes, which are connected to the Mississsippi River and the Gulf of Mexico by the Illinois River waterway.

In the 1970s, the term "water pollution" was often used to describe many of the issues in this chapter. That term has been replaced with "water quality"—yes, another politically correct "correction." So what's the definition of "good water quality?" Well, good water quality in this case means that the chemical, physical and biological integrity of the waters of the Great Lakes Basin Ecosystem is intact and not damaged. In other words, we have poor water quality in the Great Lakes Basin Ecosystem because the chemical, physical and biological integrity of the waters has been damaged, with detrimental effects on the surrounding wildlife and human life.

The Great Lakes have always raised concerns between Canada and the United States. The Boundary Waters Treaty of 1909 was created to prevent and resolve water resource disputes along the boundary between the two countries. Even as early 1909, there was a commitment not to pollute the boundary waters "to the injury of health or property on the other site."

Unfortunately, both countries broke this commitment as industry and cities built up around the Great Lakes Basin. The peak water-polluting years were between 1950 and 1975. Many of the substances polluting the Great Lakes come from the air in the form of industrial and municipal discharges that come down in the rain; sources are widespread in North America and beyond. The lakes recirculate previously deposited pollutants from cities and industries, as well. A concerted effort was made to clean up the water, and between 1972 and 1994, pollutants directly deposited into the Great Lakes were cut in half. Unfortunately, pollutants released into the air almost doubled. In Ontario, roughly 99 percent of the pollutants damaging the Great Lakes are coming from air emissions. The Canadian National Pollutant Release Inventory and the U.S. Toxics Release Inventory report similar findings, and estimate that between 73 and 85 percent of pollutants in the Great Lakes Basin are in the air (calculations vary depending on whether one is calculating on a per day basis). Factor in emissions from electric power utilities and municipal incinerators, and the air pollutants increase substantially.

1972: The Year of Watergate...and Water Quality

The first Great Lakes Water Quality Agreement was signed between Canada and the United States in 1972 (ironically to coincide with Watergate!). This was essentially a pollution control agreement between Richard Nixon and Pierre Trudeau. The good news is that today the Great Lakes Basin Ecosystem is actually cleaner than it was two decades ago. And the Canada–U.S. "clean-up team-up" does prove that governments can do something about these messes.

The bad news is that the Great Lakes were such a seething body of filth by the 1970s that, while cleaner, they're still not clean enough. We're still dealing with lingering problems, and feeling the health effects today. For example, we have not yet eliminated the persistent toxic substances that both governments agreed to eliminate back in 1978. Both countries can also jeopardize the good work that has been done through cutbacks in environmental legislation, regulation and funding for monitoring, enforcement and research.

Less than Zero
In 1995, Canadian prime minister Jean Chrétien and U.S. president Bill Clinton announced an agreement to develop a binational strategy for the virtual elimination of persistent toxic substances in the Great Lakes Basin. The two countries came up with a "target list" of chemicals, which could have promising results. "Virtual elimination" means all releases of persistent toxic chemicals due to human activity must be stopped. This hasn't happened yet. Zero discharge means no discharge of persistent toxic substances resulting from human activity. This hasn't happened yet either. In the past, these goals have been distorted to mean "less" activity or discharge by private industry. Anything less than zero is still a problem.

In the early 1990s, Lake Superior was designated a "demonstration area" for virtual elimination and zero discharge, meaning no persistent toxic substance would be permitted. Ontario, Michigan, Minnesota and Wisconsin (where Superior flows) committed to the Binational Program to Restore and Protect Lake Superior. So far, there have been "great" plans for this Great Lake, with not much action.

Great Lakes Water Quality Agreement of 1978
To meet their commitments to the water quality agreement of 1978, both the United States and Canada invested in sewage treatment facilities, stormwater runoff management, and controls for discharges coming from industry. The countries also began banning phosphorus and certain pesticides. A model water pollution control strategy comes from Ontario, through its Municipal–Industrial Strategy for Abatement (MISA), a program that works with industries such as petroleum, pulp and paper (where a lot of organochlorines come from) to control water pollution. But there are a number of activities in both countries that are reversing hard-won progress, such as:

- Relaxed pollution control policies and relaxed enforcement, including reporting and compliance requirements.
- Lack of funding and expertise for much-needed research, monitoring and enforcement. For example, the U.S. Clean Water Act is undergoing statutory review, whereby "self-audits" by various jurisdictions are being favored over federal supervision.

    We don't know enough about our Great Lakes fish, but instead of solving the problem by establishing the research resources to study the fish and learn about how toxic they are, governments, in fact, are cutting resources. For example, funds have been cut from the Great Lakes fish tissue specimen bank. This is where researchers get their fish samples so that they can monitor and assess the impact of persistent toxic chemicals on the fish. Samples are kept over the years so that comparisons can be made between, say, a millennium fish and a late 1980s fish. We need to keep this kind of research going if we want to keep eating salmon and trout. In the United States, the Agency for Toxic Substances and Disease Registry (ATSDR) may also lose funding. This is a crucial registry that studies people who consume Great Lakes fish for epidemiological studies (the study of diseases by groups of people). In other cases, enforcement responsibilities are being left to other levels of government without the resources for adequate enforcement.

- Reviews, revisions and legislative riders that weaken or even eliminate existing environmental laws. A case in point is the U.S. Toxic Substances Control Act (TSCA), originally designed to prevent additional toxic contaminants from entering the environment and to address the risks posed by existing chemicals. Approximately 72,000 chemicals are on TSCA chemicals list, but revised regulations call for a control of only 9 new chemicals in 20 years, limiting control to only polychlorinated biphenyls (PCBs). Yet there are far more toxic substances to contend with than PCBs. Similar limitations exist in Canada through the Canadian Environmental Protection Act (CEPA). This act is currently applied to a relatively small number of listed substances, using the chemical-by-chemical approach instead of the class-of-chemicals approach.

Worst Areas

The Great Lakes Basin is divided into Areas of Concern and Areas of Quality. Areas of Concern include Toronto Bay (which may be the next Olympics site), Hamilton Harbor, Green Bay–Fox River, Duluth, Minnesota, and Ashtabula, Ohio. Collingwood, Ontario, was delisted as an Area of Concern in the mid-1990s. Altogether, there are 43 Areas of Concern. **171**

Areas are ranked by how many species are declining or living in degraded conditions, whether the nutrients in the area are in good or bad shape, and how many contaminants are affecting wildlife and human health. For example, phosphorus was once a huge problem, but sewage treatment plant upgrades have taken care of it. To date, many Areas of Concern are due for upgrades, and haven't had them yet.

A CATALOGUE OF PROBLEMS

Anyone living in the Great Lakes Basin depends upon its ecosystem for drinking water and fresh fish. As explained earlier, persistent toxic substances are largely organochlorines, a class of toxins that include pesticides and PCBs, dioxins, furans and similar substances, which break down into an estrogen-like substance that is being linked to a host of estrogenic cancers, as well as to poor sperm counts and hermaphroditic traits in many fish and wildlife species.

In the 1980s, many Great Lakes fisheries were closed down because dangerous substances such as mercury and PCBs were found in lake trout and salmon. In the mid-1990s, a retrospective risk assessment suggested that dioxin in Lake Ontario may have caused complete reproductive failure in native lake trout populations in the early 1940s. Today, lake trout is usually produced through fish farming, known as "artificial stocking," which hasn't proved to be the best alternative (trout prefer their natural habitat). As you may recall from chapter 8, food contamination has far-reaching social consequences, too. Contamination of perch, the dietary staple on the Akwesasne Reserve, led to widespread chronic health problems among the residents there.

These toxins are not limited to the Great Lakes, however. For example, pesticides were found in a lake on Isle Royale at concentrations higher than those in the surrounding waters of Lake Superior. They've also been found in Florida, the Netherlands and the Arctic. It is a global problem that is magnified in the Great Lakes Basin. In its last three Biennial Reports, the International Joint Commission provided more than 50 recommendations that involved toxic and persistent toxic substances.

Who's Most at Risk for Great Lakes Health Problems?

Some people are more at risk for Great Lakes health problems than others:

- People who consume a large amount of Great Lakes fish. Those at greatest risk for health problems are those who consume fish they have caught themselves (people who fish for livelihood or sport). Aside from sport fishermen, people who depend on catching their own fish to survive are often poor, with no access to "safe fish" that has passed inspection by fisheries (which actually may not mean much, as you'll read below). Native peoples are particularly at risk for consuming toxic sport fish and game that are fish-eating. There are roughly 63 native Canadian communities in the northern part of the Great Lakes Basin, where some of the worst contaminants are. You can purchase the government of Canada's Guide to Eating Ontario Sport Fish (1997, 1998) by calling 1-800-820-2716.

- Fetuses. When exposed to toxic chemicals in utero, fetuses can be born with developmental disabilities as well as reproductive health problems, such as undescended testicles. One study involved human infants in upper New York State whose mothers ate Lake Ontario salmon prior to pregnancy. The findings (reported in 1995) suggest that behavioral abnormalities are more prevalent in the babies born to this group of women. And, in fact, the same behavioral abnormalities were found 15 years ago in babies born to a group of mothers who ate Lake Michigan fish.
- Breastfed children. Again, breast milk can pass on levels of toxins that exceed guidelines for human health.
- People who drink untreated water in the Great Lakes Basin. Members of this group are exposing themselves to a host of bacterial, viral and protozoan contamination, which can lead to gastrointestinal illnesses.
- People who swim in these waters. They are at risk of contamination through swallowing water, or skin exposure—bathing, boating or other water sports on the Great Lakes can increase exposure to toxins.

Sources of Priority Contaminants and Routes of Exposure

Source: *Great Lakes Health Effects Program 1993.*

Radioactive Substances

Where there is lots of water, there are lots of nuclear power stations! And that means there is concern about the potential for nuclear accidents and core water being dumped into the lakes; there is concern about production,

Contaminant	Sources	Routes of Human Exposure
Polychlorinated Biphenyls (PCBs)	Used in electrical transformers and capacitors, and in hydraulic equipment; also as lubricants and heat-transfer fluids. Released to environment primarily from equipment in use and by waste site leakage.	Consumption of contaminated foods, particularly fish, meat, and dairy products.
Polychlorinated dibenzo-*p*-dioxins (PCDDs) (esp. 2,3,7,8-TCDD) an dipolychlorinated dibenzofurans (PCDFs)	Formed as impurities during the synthesis of various chlorinated compounds (e.g., certain pesticides and herbicides); released through pulp and paper bleaching and solid waste incineration; found in exhaust from vehicles using fossil fuels; and can also result from the combustion of any chlorinated organic material.	Consumption of contaminated foods, particularly fish, meat, and dairy products.
Dichlorodiphenyl trichloroethane (DDT) and its degradation products (e.g., DDE)	An insecticide now banned in Canada and the U.S. Sources are leakage from waste sites and atmospheric transport and deposition.	Consumption of contaminated foods, especially fish and dairy products.
Mirex	A fire retardant and contact insecticide once used in Canada and the U.S. but now banned. Extremely persistent; may reach the GLB via surface run-off from contaminated soils or by leaching from hazardous waste sites.	Consumption of contaminated foods.
Toxaphene	An insecticide used on cotton fields. Its use is restricted in Canada and the U.S. Sources include contaminated soils, hazardous waste sites, and air transport.	Consumption of contaminated foods.
Aldrin and Dieldrin (i.e., chlorinated cyclodienes. Other examples are chlordane and its metabolites, heptachlor and heptachlor epoxide)	Aldrin and dieldrin are insecticides used for control of soil insects and mosquitoes. Dieldrin is also produced from the metabolic oxidation of aldrin. Their use is restricted.	Consumption of contaminated foods, especially fish.
Hexachlorobenzene (HCB)	A fungicide no longer used in Canada or the U.S.; also generated as a by-product of fuel combustion and the production of some pesticides.	Consumption of contaminated foods, especially fish.
Hexachlorocyclohexanes	An insecticide, lindane is one of	

(HCHs) (e.g., lindane)	8 HCH isomers. HCH is the key isomer found in human tissue, accumulating in body fat. No longer produced in the U.S., but still in use as an import. Registered for use in Alberta.	Consumption of contaminated foods. Can be transported by water and air.
Microbial Contaminants (e.g., bacteria, viruses, protozoa)	Found in poorly treated sewage discharge, agricultural run-off and urban run-off; also storm water run-off, animal feces.	Consumption of contaminated drinking water or recreational water; absorption through breaks in the skin.
Radionuclides	Natural radiation comes primarily from radioactive elements in the earth's crust, with additional but minor contributions from cosmic rays and cosmogenic radionuclides. Anthropogenic sources include nuclear weapons test fallout and emissions from nuclear fuel cycle operations.	Inhalation of contaminated air and consumption of contaminated food and water (internal dosing), and exposure by direct irradiation (external dosing).
Methylmercury (MeHg)	Biosynthesis as result of atmospheric deposition of elemental mercury from natural oceanic output (30–40% of annual Hg emissions to atmosphere); released from inundated vegetation. Inorganic Hg occurs naturally in soils and as a by-product of chlor-alkali, paint, and electrical equipment production processes. MeHg bioconcentrates in fish.	Consumption of contaminated fish and marine products.
Cadmium	Waste dumps and waste incinerators, fertilizers, sewage sludge, solid wastes, cadmium mining/refining operations, soil, plant-life, atmospheric deposition.	Consumption of contaminated foods, esp. organ meats (liver, kidney), seafood (shellfish, crustaceans), and cereals (e.g., wild rice); tobacco use; consumption of drinking water (minor).
Lead	Combustion of leaded gasoline, metal smelters, automotive batteries, contaminated soil and dust, lead-based paints, drinking water in contact with lead-soldered pipes, atmospheric deposition.	In the absence of a point source of contamination, consumption of contaminated foods and drinking water; inhalation of contaminated air.
Ground-level Ozone	Formed from the interaction of nitrogren oxides and hydrocarbons in the atmosphere in presence of sunlight. Can be transported long distances.	Inhalation of contaminated air.
Acid Aerosols	Formed when pollutants such as sulphur dioxide and oxides	Inhalation of contaminated

Airborne particles	of nitrogen are transformed in the atmosphere in the presence of sunlight; may be transported long distances from original source in the form of rain, snow, vapor, fine particles and gases; can be both air and water pollutants.	air.
Polycyclic Aromatic Hydrocarbons (PAHs) (e.g., benzo[a]pyrene)	Very small pieces of solid or liquid matter that vary in size, chemical composition and source. Can be coarse or fine. Fine particles arise mainly from man-made sources such as combustion of fuels, and include sulphates and nitrates as well as metals. Coarse particles consist largely of naturally occurring substances, particularly soil.	Inhalation of contaminated air.
Volatile Organic Compounds (VOCs) (e.g., trihalomethanes, benzene, trichloroethylene)	Incomplete combustion of fossil fuels, organic matter, and solid waste; combustion activities associated with industry (e.g., coke production, metal smelting, oil refining). Non-commercial sources include wood-burning fireplaces, cigarette smoke, vehicle exhaust; and smoked, grilled, fried, or barbecued meat and fish.	Inhalation of contaminated air and consumption of certain foods.
	Formed from natural or industrial sources by the interaction of chlorine with organic materials; also found in dry-cleaning solvents; both an airborne and drinking water contaminant.	Inhalation of contaminated air from exposure to chlorinated tap water during showering, bathing or to dry-cleaning solvents, and consumption of drinking water.

use and storage of radioactive materials and nuclear wastes, as well as what to do about *decommissioned* nuclear power stations. Radioactive materials get discharged into the Great Lakes and affect our health, which can lead to

Routes of Contamination

How do contaminants from the Great Lakes get into our bodies? Here are all the ways it can happen:

- Food and fish. While Michigan fish advisories may ban one kind of toxic fish, Ontario fish advisories may allow the sale of that same fish. So the first order of business is for all eight Great Lakes states and Ontario to agree on which fish to ban, and which fish to sell.
- Drinking water
- Milk
- Our skin (through dermal exposure)
- Inhalation

Tests done on bodily secretions and excretions (urine, feces, saliva, breast milk, sweat) have confirmed the presence of toxins from all of these sources; additional tests on hair samples have also added verification.

When you mix airborne contaminants with the "lake effect" winds, it contributes to ozone depletion, smog, and "acid rain," which gets directly into our crops and other vegetation—and then hits the food chain.

a number of cancers. But the problem is that there is no comprehensive

Climate Changes

In early December 1999, while most Great Lakes residents were enjoying temperatures of close to 20 degrees Celsius, I was feeling that something was wrong with the state of the universe. While out and about doing my holiday shopping, I heard many retailers and passersby volunteer their discomfort with the "unusually warm weather" we were having for that time of year. And rightly so! One of the most serious ozone issues is how climate in the Great Lakes Basin is affected.

Many experts predict that the Great Lakes climate will become warmer and drier, resulting in decreased water levels, which means less water for the forests and wetlands upon which many wildlife species depend. Our terrain may change as a result, and we will see more exotic species of fish, animals and plants and less species native to the Great Lakes Basin.

A drier climate will also make it necessary for Great Lakes businesses and residents to conserve water. This heavily settled and industrialized area is currently one of the highest per capita consumers of water in the world, but increased water (and related energy) costs will make the area less attractive to live and work in.

inventory of how many radioactive substances are released around the

Great Lakes Basin.

WHAT TO REQUEST FROM THE GREAT LAKES BUSINESS COMMUNITY

Many of the suggestions made in chapters 7 and 8 for getting businesses—primarily industry—on board with stopping cancer at the source programs are relevant here, too, as we're dealing with the same issues: trying to eliminate airborne toxins and persistent toxic substances, while stopping the release of any new substance until it's been proven safe. In addition, it's

Other Great Lakes Problems

Cancer increases notwithstanding, here are some other serious problems in the Great Lakes Basin.

Natural Habitat

We need to save the Great Lakes natural habitat, and need to have healthy plant life to support its aquatic life and wetlands creatures. At least 14 species of fish and fish-eating wildlife in the region suffer from serious reproductive problems. Programs such as Partners for Wildlife in the United States, and the North American Wildlife Management Plan and the Fish and Wildlife Restoration Project in Hamilton Harbor, Canada, are making a good start in focusing on Great Lakes habitat issues. Even so, the U.S. Fish and Wildlife Service has listed 22 endangered and/or threatened species in the Great Lakes that are affected by poor water quality. According to Environment Canada reports, the entire shorelines of Lake Ontario, Lake Erie and southern Lake Huron are destroying numerous species due to pesticide use by agriculture. Even with various programs in place, both the Canadian and U.S. governments are starting to have more relaxed standards for habitat protection.

Biocontamination

Biocontamination occurs when non-native wildlife or plant species are introduced into a new area, destroying or interfering with native wildlife or plant species. Over the last hundred years, roughly 140 non-native or exotic species have been introduced into the Great Lakes region, which include the infamous purple loosestrife (a colorful weed that wreaks havoc with other plant life), as well as the zebra mussel. Zebra mussels caused the extinction of native clams in Lake Erie in less than a decade. As a result, smelt and yellow and white perch are now endangered species.

Non-native species come from ships and unwittingly stow away as water from one region gets shipped into other waters (called ballast water). This is how young flounder got into Thunder Bay and Lake Erie. By pumping out ballast water before the ship's old water is introduced into new water, we can control this growing problem. And again, climate changes are starting to make the Great Lakes Basin attractive to more exotic species.

Lake Ontario Biomagnification of PCBs
As PCBs work their way up the food chain, their concentrations in animal tissue can be magnified up to 25 million times. Microscopic organisms pick up persistent chemicals from sediments (a continuing source of contamination) and water, and are consumed in large numbers by filter-feeding tiny animals called zooplankton. Larger species like mysids then consume zooplankton, fish eat the mysids, and so on up the food chain to the herring gull.

important to contact local businesses and insist they be aware of the environmental practices of anyone they are partnering with outside of Canada and/or the United States. When we import contaminated products from other countries, we contaminate our own country. There are also some specific requests we must make of Great Lakes businesses and industries:

- Alternatives to polyvinyl chloride (PVC), which is mostly manufactured and used in the Great Lakes Basin, must be found. Currently, the industry states that its production and use is harmless and even environmentally beneficial, that PVC is a stable product and its manufacture does not cause pollution. But experts are concerned about PVC's eventual disposal and destruction through incineration or the open environment.

- Encourage small businesses to get themselves included in the general cleanup programs. Small businesses are often missed by government programs and trade associations. The dry-cleaning industry, for example, uses solvents that pose a hazard to the environment, to customers and employees. Other small industries include the printing and graphic arts industry, automotive products, auto body repair, the manufacture and installation of floor coverings, photography labs and machine components. Pay attention to what kinds of illnesses are prevalent in different businesses. If stats aren't kept, find out why not. Alternative processes are imperative, and can be developed if enough consumers, like you and me, complain. Small businesses can be supported through government incentive programs or grants to retrofit (upgrade) to environmentally sound processes.

- Businesses large and small, plus their customers (that's us) must support one another in purchasing environmentally friendly products.
- All businesses should produce separate environmental annual reports that provide public accountability regarding how they are contributing to virtual elimination and zero discharge.

Fishing for Funding

One of the most natural places to go for funding Great Lakes Basin cleanup programs of any sort is fish-related industries. A letter requesting funding or volunteers from any of the following businesses, with a reminder of how they can capitalize on the good PR a cleanup program will generate, is an excellent start. These businesses can also join in partnership with government to help fund educational initiatives:

- Frozen-fish food manufacturers
- Fish/seafood restaurants
- Fishing-supplies companies, retailers or manufacturers
- Hotel and tourism industries that specialize in boating or fishing sports
- Boating manufacturers
- Water-sports manufacturers

WHAT TO RECOMMEND TO YOUR GREAT LAKES GOVERNMENT

Once again, it's up to you and I to lobby our local governments for the following:

- Funding for continued enforcement of the Great Lakes Water Quality Agreement and other pro-environmental policies in the Great Lakes Basin. The trend has been to cut funding rather than provide it, and we want to see this trend reversed. To obtain a copy of the Great Lakes Water Quality Agreement, visit *www.great-lakes.net*. Lakewide Management Plans (LAMPS) are local programs that focus on specific areas in the Great Lakes Basin that can really help to police certain areas and enforce aspects of the Great Lakes Water Quality Agreement. Experts have been recommending LAMPS for years, but so far there is a lack of funding and action to get them started.
- Funding and programs to restore Areas of Concern. If Collingwood, Ontario, can be restored and delisted as an Area of Concern, so can other areas in the Great Lakes Basin.

- Health Risk Education programs for Great Lakes residents, particularly for citizens in Areas of Concern. We need to be informed of the health risks we are facing so that we can make healthier lifestyle choices, and perhaps go for regular screenings for at-risk cancers.
- Education for health care providers (especially in Areas of Concern) so that they can help to validate complaints of ill health, and be more prudent in referring people for regular screening for certain cancers that are more prevalent in those areas. This entails support from universities, environmental health chairs in professional schools of health sciences, research and teaching hospitals, and related businesses, such as the pharmaceutical industry. We need more health care practitioners who are informed, up-to-date and knowledgeable about environmental medicine. Round tables and workshops need to be coordinated along with support from the Canadian Great Lakes Health Effects Program and the U.S. Agency for Toxic Substances and Disease Registry (ATSDR).
- The establishment of Environmental Health as a credible profession to attract young doctors to specialize and train in it. Trust me—we're going to need these kinds of professionals in droves, and already there is a serious shortage.
- Fishing education programs to warn people who sport-fish of the dangers of contaminants and the routes of fish contamination. These programs can also include labels that identify risky fish so that we can choose other foods.
- A list of known pollutants coming into the Great Lakes Basin from both Canada and the United States for constituents and consumers.
- More research programs to examine toxins in the Great Lakes Basin and how they affect our health. Areas that desperately need to be researched are human health effects, water conservation (it's coming!) and cleanup technologies in Areas of Concern. Again, universities and private business can help to fund research.
- A reduction in incineration. Again, a lot of water pollutants start in the air, particularly through municipal, industrial and medical/hospital incinerators. Right now, waste management programs allow and even encourage incineration. Although newly upgraded incinerators are okayed by governments, the results are not okay. We need alternatives to incineration if we want to reduce pollutants in the Great Lakes Basin.
- A decrease in mercury. Mercury mainly comes from thermal power stations. We need to find ways of reducing mercury emissions, which have

serious health consequences.

Cleaning up the Great Lakes is a long process, and a long time coming, but we cannot deny the increased cancer risks and other health problems in the Great Lakes Basin. In the 1980s, we all learned the 3 R's (Reduce, Reuse and Recycle) to help reduce the amount of garbage being poured into landfill sites. In the new millennium, we need to learn two P's: Precaution (proving a chemical is safe before use instead of proving it guilty later) and Phase Out By Class (pulling categories of chemicals "from the shelves," not just single chemicals).

In the 1980s, 11 critical pollutants were identified by the Great Lakes Water Quality Board: PCBs, DDT and its metabolites, dieldrin, toxaphene, mirex, dioxin, furans, benzopyrene and hexachlorobenzene, lead and mercury. Health Canada also identified radionuclides, airborne contaminants and micro-organisms as problematic. Many of these substances are still not gone, are still being produced, and are waiting for their final sunset. And in the meantime, there are several hundred contaminants in the Great Lakes Basin that freely persist.

Part III
PUTTING IT ALL TOGETHER

As you can see, there are a variety of behaviors that fall into the category of "What's Personal" (chapters 2 through 6)—personal lifestyle habits that can be modified to help stop cancer at the source. Then there are the environmental exposures that fall into the category of "What's Political" (chapters 7 through 9). These are exposures to carcinogenic substances that are beyond our personal control today, but definitely within our collective control for the future. By raising our collective voices of concern and protest, we can definitely help to change the state of the earth, and stop cancer at the source in our descendants.

Cancer rates among North American children under the age of 15 have increased by roughly 25 percent within the last 25 years; the highest rates of childhood cancer are seen in children under age 5. Cancer is considered to be the second major cause of death in children after accidents.

> The lifestyle of toddlers has not changed much over the past half century. Young children do not smoke, drink alcohol or hold stressful jobs. Children do, however, receive a greater dose of whatever chemicals are in the air, food and water because, pound for pound, they breathe, eat and drink more than adults do.
> —Sandra Steingraber, *Living Downstream* (1997, Addison-Wesley: 39)

10

STOPPING CANCER AT THE SOURCE: PROGRAMS AND ACTION PLANS

This chapter is an overview of how to put a lot of the "What's Political" information into action.

In 2001 and beyond, more North Americans will die of cancer than ever before; cancer deaths increased by more than 20 percent in the 1990s. In 1998, a man's lifetime risk of developing cancer was 40.9 percent; his lifetime risk of dying from the disease was 26.9 percent. In 1998, a woman had a 35 percent chance of developing cancer and a 22.4 percent chance of dying from it. Just to give you an idea of the seriousness of this statistic, in the 1930s, one in ten people developed cancer. By the 1970s, it was one in five; today it is one in two. This is alarming news in light of the fact that our risks for many cancers increase as we age. In 1994, 33 million North Americans were over age 65. Now, more than 100 million North Americans are over 65. And by the year 2010, the growth rate of the older population will be three and a half times as high as that of the total population.

Today, cancer is "controlled" through early detection, treatment, rehabilitation and palliative care (which means symptom relief rather than curative treatment). These are not great ways to ultimately deal with the problem of cancer. We really need to stop the disease at the source, which is what we do with an infinite variety of diseases ranging from heart disease to AIDS. This is not to say that we should abandon research into new treatments, but that we must also look at what, in our behavior or environment, can change to reduce cancer incidence.

Not all cancers are on the rise, however. We are beginning to see a reduction in the incidence and mortality of a few major cancers, including lung cancer in men, and stomach and colorectal cancer in both sexes. No one knows why we're seeing a decline in stomach cancer. (Forty-six years ago, stomach cancer was the most worrisome cancer in the world, and it has now fallen to eleventh place in North America for both sexes combined, due in large part to a decline in the consumption of preserved or pickled foods.) But the decline in lung cancer in men and colon cancer in both sexes is attributed to more aggressive anti-smoking campaigns as well as better education about fiber and high-fiber diets.

Since so many cancers are linked to poor diet and sedentary living, by focusing on anticancer programs aimed at stopping cancer at the source, we can also help reduce the incidence of a number of the killer chronic diseases, such as heart disease or Type 2 diabetes. By looking at environmental toxins, we may also be able to reduce the incidence of more mysterious environmental diseases, such as chronic fatigue syndrome (CFS) or multiple chemical sensitivity (MCS).

The people who will benefit most from stopping cancer at the source programs are your children and grandchildren. In order to prevent future cancer, we have to look at its natural history. Many cancers (including breast and stomach cancer) are influenced by events in childhood as well as later in life. Strategies we adopt today may take 20 to 40 years to deliver a clear return or benefit. This is one of the reasons that it's been so difficult to convince governments to spend money on stopping cancer at the source programs, and why the bulk of research is going into more "tangible" areas, such as treatment or the identification of cancer genes. But that doesn't mean that delaying these initiatives makes sense; it means that the sooner we act, the sooner we can see the rewards.

WHAT GOVERNMENT CAN DO

In order for a stopping cancer at the source program to work, you have to have some form of government on your side, be it municipal/civic, provincial/state or federal. Although most health promotion experts agree that cancer prevention is a population-by-population issue, it is the higher levels of government that control the policy "levers" and funds needed to bring about meaningful change. But with the proper funding and support, stopping cancer at the source programs can be led by public health units and community initiatives. Cancer prevention, insofar as it is population-based, appears to be a provincial or state responsibility, rather than a federal one. One kind of cancer may be more common in one region and less common in another, for example.

Stopping cancer at the source programs also have to be tackled from both the community and individual level. That means that while only you can choose not to smoke, the government can help you make that choice by passing laws that will make it more difficult for you to obtain or afford cigarettes, or ban certain kinds of advertising that may entice you into smoking, or ban smoking in public places. In other words, the goal of stopping cancer at the source programs is to spend money on maintaining and enhancing good health, rather than pouring all health money into treating and rehabilitating people already in poor health. Ideally, the money should be allocated to the front and back equally or, at least, appropriately. So what all this boils down to is educating the public about ways to change diet, lifestyle and certain behaviors that can cause certain cancers, and then backing up that education with policies or laws that can help people implement those changes. For example, it is difficult for people living in northern regions to adopt a high-fiber, low-fat diet, avoid exposure to cancer-causing chemicals or eat organically grown produce when there is no access to fresh produce or the kinds of healthy foods they are encouraged to eat. In other words, you can stop using cancer-causing pesticides on your own lawn, but you need government to decide not to spray the park or school grounds where your children play.

What and Who is Involved?

Good stopping cancer at the source strategies and programs are really large-scale projects that involve health professions, business, advocacy groups and non-governmental organizations such as the Canadian Cancer Society or the National Cancer Institute. Clearly, this takes coordination; one idea public health experts favor is adopting "stop cancer" networks, which would enforce various policies or recommendations. These could include representatives from all areas, such as health, labor, business advocacy and consumer groups. And while you might think that the Department or Ministry of Health ought to "run the show," stopping cancer at the source programs will need all the other departments/ministries to participate, such as Education, Environment, Agriculture, Food and Rural Affairs.

Here are just a few things we need a stopping cancer at the source network to do:

- Develop and coordinate education campaigns and "backup" policies;
- Identify the barriers to stopping cancer education and policies;
- Come up with ways to overcome these barriers;

- Coordinate educational programs; and
- Form coalitions addressing cancer-related risk factors at the community level.

How Do You Educate the Public?

Educating the public involves using the media. Television, the Internet, radio, magazine and newspaper articles and targeted print literature, such as posters and pamphlets, are one way. But there are other ways to get the message out:

- Training health professionals to provide counseling on smoking cessation and the risks associated with exposure to environmental tobacco smoke;
- Offering workshops on healthy food preparation and shopping skills;
- Maintaining current efforts to promote and protect employees' "right to know" about hazardous substances in the workplace (as well as citizens' right to know about cancer risks in their community); and
- Adopting public education initiatives to increase awareness of environmental health risks.

The right education programs should encourage us to make healthy and *informed* choices not just by raising our awareness, but by changing our attitudes about our health and well being. For example, education may not reduce the levels of hazardous chemicals in somebody's workplace; but awareness that those hazardous chemicals exist may change somebody's decision about whether to work in that hazardous environment or to find alternative, less hazardous substances that can be substituted.

"Walking the Talk"

Educating the public on what can cause cancer means backing up the education with the programs and legislation that can facilitate the now-educated public to make healthier choices and/or reduce their exposure to carcinogenic substances. Examples of healthy policies include:

- Making it easier to adopt healthy living practices. That means making healthy food available to all regions and creating smoke-free workplaces and public places, including restaurants.
- Making it more difficult to add unhealthy living practices to our current lifestyle. For example, this could mean "sin taxes" on cigarettes or junk foods.
- Creating healthy physical and social environments. Creating public,

free access to outdoor "green spaces" (parks, etc.) and sufficient indoor recreational spaces or programs will help people get "out there."

Actual legislation might include:

- High tobacco taxes;
- Banning smoking in the workplace;
- Developing a food labeling system that is both nutritionally informative and consumer-friendly;
- Making sure healthy school breakfast and lunch programs are available to all children who need them;
- Setting realistic and measurable timetables for the sunsetting of persistent toxic substances that are known or suspected carcinogens; and
- Instituting gasoline vapor recovery programs at all fuel transfer facilities and gas stations in order to reduce our exposure to carcinogenic emissions.

The following are just a few examples of environmentally friendly policies or legislation that help stop cancer at the source:

- Smoke-free public places (including restaurants and bars);
- The ban on tobacco sales to minors;
- Healthy food alternatives in school and workplace cafeterias;
- Income that allows for the purchase of nutritious food;
- Workplaces free from dangerous levels of occupational carcinogens; and
- Pollution-free soil, air and drinking water.

You can help make stopping cancer at the source programs work with your consumer power. All of the unknown carcinogens to which we may be exposed through the air, water and food chain can slowly be dealt with through collective efforts. Call, fax, email and write as this book suggests. Use your consumer lobbying powers to save your children, this planet and maybe yourself. There are dozens of ways in which you can use your consumer and constituent powers. If every reader tried just one, we would be much further ahead than we are today in stopping cancer at the source.

APPENDIX A
RESOURCE LIST

IN THE UNITED STATES

International Joint Commission offices:
1250-23rd Street NW, Suite 100
Washington, D.C. 20440
202-736-9000
100 Metcalfe Street, 18th Floor
Ottawa, Ontario K1P 5M1
613-995-2984

The U.S. Department of Health and Human Services
200 Independence Avenue, SW
Washington, D.C. 20201
202-619-0257
Toll Free: 1-877-696-6775
www.hhs.gov

National Cancer Institute
NCI Public Inquiries Office
Building, 31, Room 10A03
31 Center Drive, MSC 2580
BETHESDA, MD 20892-2580
301-435-3848
www.nci.nih.gov

The Center for Nutrition Policy and Promotion
1120 20th Street, NW, Suite 200, North Lobby,
Washington, D.C. 20036,
Telephone: 202-418-2312, Fax: 202-208-2321.
www.usda.gov/cnpp

National Food Safety Database
(U.S. Department of Agriculture)
University of Florida
Old Dairy Science Building
120, Room 105
Box 110365
Gainesville, Fl 32611-0365
www.foodsafety.org

Organic Trade Association (serving North America)
50 Miles Street
P.O. Box 1078
Greenfield, MA 01302
413-774-7511
www.ota.com

The Organic Consumers Association
6101 Cliff Estate Rd
Little Marais, MN 55614
Telephone: 218-226-4164, Fax: 218-226-4157
www.purefood.org

Working Group on Community Right-To-Know
218 D Street SE
Washingon, D.C. 20003
202-544-9586
www.rtk.net/wcs

Right-to-Know Network at the Unison Institute
1731 Connecticut Avenue NW
Washington, D.C. 20009
202-234-8494

Children's Environmental Health Network
5900 Hollis Street, Suite R3
Emeryville, CA 94608
Telephone: 510-597-1393
Fax: 510-597-1399
Email: cehn@cehn.org
www.cehn.org

The John Snow Institute's Center for Environmental Health Studies
44 Farnsworth Street
Boston, MA 02210
617-482-9485

Center for Health, Environment and Justice
P.O. Box 6806
Falls Church, VA 22040
703-237-2249
www.chej.org/about.html

Environmental Research Foundation
P.O. Box 5036
Annapolis, MD 21403
410-263-1584
www.rachel.org

Environmental Protection Agency
401 M Street SW
Washington, D.C. 20460
Hotline: 800-535-0202
www.epa.gov
(to obtain a copy of the Toxics Release Inventory)
For information on hazardous waste: 800-424-9346
For information on water contamination: 800-426-4791
For information on health effects of environmental contaminants:
202-260-1023

U.S. Agency for Toxic Substances and Disease Registry
1600 Clifton Road NE
Atlanta, GA 30333

404-639-0501
www.atsdr.cdc.gov

The Clearinghouse on Environmental Health Effects
Hotline: 800-643-4794
www.infoventures.com/e-hlth
(this service provided by the National Institute of Environmental Health Sciences)

National Coalition Against the Misuse of Pesticides
701 E Street SE, Suite 200
Washington, D.C. 20003
202-543-5450
www.ncamp.org

The Northwest Coalition For Alternatives To Pesticides
P.O. Box 1393
Eugene, OR 97440
541-344-5044
www.efn.org/~ncap

The Pesticide Action Network North American Regional Center
116 New Montgomery Street, Suite 810
San Francisco, CA 94104
415-541-9140
www.panna.org

Pesticide Education Center
P.O. Box 420870
San Francisco, CA 94142
415-391-8511
www.igc.org/pesticides

Rachel Carson Council
8940 Jones Mill Road
Chevy Chase, MD 20815
301-652-1877
www.members.aol.com/rccouncil/ourpage

Breast Cancer and Environmental Risk Factors Project
(searchable database on breast cancer and environmental risk factors)
www.cfe.cornell.edu/bcerf

IN CANADA

Canadian Autoworkers' (CAW) Health and Safety Department
205 Placer Court
Toronto, ON M2H 3H9
416-495-6558 or 1-800-268-5763
Fax: 416-495-6554
www.caw.ca

Canadian Centre for Occupational Health and Safety
250 Main Street East
Hamilton, ON
L8N 1H6
1-800-263-8466
(toll-free in Canada)
1-905-572-4400 (8:30 AM to 5:00 PM Eastern Time)
1-905-572-4500 (FAX)
www.ccohs.ca

National Pollutant Release Inventory (a guide to access-to-information
laws) available through: Information Commissioner of Canada
112 Kent Street
Ottawa, ON K1A 1H3
1-800-267-0441
www.ec.gc.ca/pdb/npri

Canadian Centre for Pollution Prevention
100 Charlotte Street,
Sarnia, ON N7T 4R2
1-800-667-9790
www.C2P2online.com

Democracy Watch
P.O. Box 821 Station B
Ottawa, ON K1P 5P9

613-241-5179
www.dwatch.ca

Canadian Environmental Law Association
517 College Street, Suite 401
Toronto, ON M6G 4A2
416-960-2284
www.cela.ca

The Canadian Cancer Registry
Health Canada
Tunney's Pasture
Ottawa, ON K1A 0L2
613-957-0327
www.cihi.ca/Roadmap/Cancer

Canadian Organic Growers Association
The National Information Network for Organic Farmers, Gardeners and
Consumers
Toll free phone: 1-877-677-6055
Local phone: 1-613-767-0796
Fax: 1-613-757-1291
Email: pbenner@webhart.net
www.cog.ca

Canada's Food Guide to Healthy Eating
For copies of this brochure, contact:
Publications Health Canada
Ottawa, ON K1A 0K9
613-954-5995
www.hc-sc.gc.ca/hppb/nutrition/pube/foodguid

Bibliography

Primary Sources

Note: the following sources were used to compile the Ontario Task Force Report On The Primary Prevention of Cancer, released March 1995.

Accelerated Reduction/Elimination Toxics. ARET Candidate Substances List. Hull, Quebec: ARET, 1994.

Advisory Committee on Environmental Standards. A Standard for Tritium: A Recommendation to the Minister of Environment and Energy. Toronto: ACES Report 94-01, 1994.

Agriculture Canada. Ontario farm groundwater quality survey. Summer 1992. ISBN 0-662-20879-X. Ottawa, 1993.

Alavanja, M.C.R., R.C. Brownson, J.L. Lubin, et al. "Residential radon exposure and lung cancer among nonsmoking women." *J Natl Cancer Inst* 1994; 86: 1829-1837.

Bates, D., and R. Sitzo. "Air pollution and hospital admissions in Southern Ontario: the acid summer haze effect." *Environmental Research* 1987; 4: 203-22.

Barker, D.J.P., et al. "Poor housing in childhood and high rates of stomach cancer in England and Wales." *Br J Cancer* 1990; 61: 675-678.

Beral, V., and N. Robinson. "The relationship of malignant melanoma, basal and squamous skin cancers to indoor and outdoor work." *Br J Cancer* 1981; 44: 886-892.

Bergkvist, L.H.O. Adami, I. Persson, R. Hoover, and C. Schairer. "The risk of breast cancer after estrogen and estrogen-progestin replacement." *New Eng J Med* 1989; 321: 293-297.

Black, D., et al. The Black Report (Report of the Working Group on Inequalities in Health). London: DHSS, 1980.

Cancer 2000 Task Force Inequalities in Cancer Control in Canada. Ottawa: Cancer 2000 Task Force Panel on Cancer and the Disadvantaged, 1992.

Carlson, C. "A comprehensive school-based substance abuse program with cooperative community involvement." *J Primary Prevention* 1990; 10: 289-302.

Carmichael, J.A., and P.D. Maskens. "Cervical dysplasia and human papillomavirus." *Am J Obstet Gynecol* 1989; 160: 916-918.

Caygill, C.P., et al. "Occupational and socioeconomic factors associated with peptic ulcer and with cancers following consequent gastric surgery." *Ann Occ Hyg* 1990; 34: 19-27.

CDC (Centers for Disease Control) "Cancer and steroid hormone study. Combination oral contraceptives use and the risk of ovarian cancer." *JAMA* 1983; 249: 1596-1599.

————. "Cancer and steroid hormone study. Combination oral contraceptives use and the risk of ovarian cancer." *JAMA* 1987; 257: 796-800.

Chief Medical Officer of Health. Progress Against Cancer. Toronto, Ministry of Health, Ontario, 1994.

Colborne, T., and C. Clement. *Chemically-Induced Alterations in Sexual Functioning and Development: The Wildlife-Human Connection.* Princeton, New Jersey: Princeton Scientific Publishing Co., 1992.

Committee on Diet and Health. Diet and Health. Implications for reducing chronic disease risk. Washington D.C., National Academy Press, 1989.

Cooke, K.R., D.C.G. Skegg, and J. Fraser. "Socio-economic status, indoor and outdoor work and malignant melanoma." *Int J Cancer* 1984; 37: 57-62.

Council on Scientific Affairs. "Cancer risk of pesticides in agricultural workers." *JAMA* 1988; 260: 959-966.

Daling, J.R., K.E. Malone, L.F. Voigt, et al. "Risk of breast cancer among young women: relationship to induced abortion. *J Natl Cancer Inst* 1994; 86: 1584-1592.

Davies, K. "Human exposure routes to selected persistent toxic chemicals in the Great Lakes Basin." Toronto: City of Toronto Dept Pub Hlth, 1986.

————. "Concentrations and dietary intake of selected organochlorines, including PCBs, PCDDs and PCDFs in fresh food composites grown in Ontario, Canada." *Chemosphere* 1988; 17: 263-276.

Davies, D.L., A. Blair, and D.G. Hoel. "Agricultural exposures and cancer trends in developed countries." *Envir Health Perspectives* 1992; 100: 39-44.

Davies, D.L., et al. "Medical hypothesis: xenoestrogens as preventable causes of breast cancer." *Envir Health Perspectives* 1993; 101: 372-377.

Dewailly, E., S. Dodin, R. Verault, et al. "High organochlorine body burden in women with estrogen receptor-positive breast cancer" (brief communication). *J Natl Cancer Institute* 1994; 86: 232-234.

Doll, R., and R. Peto. "The causes of cancer: quantitative estimates of avoidable risks of cancer in the United States today." *J Natl Cancer Institute* 1981; 66: 1191-1308.

Edwards, G. *Alcohol Policy and the Public Good*. Oxford: Oxford University Press, 1994.

Ekbom, A., et al. "Evidence of prenatal influences on breast cancer." *Lancet* 1992; 340, 1015-1018.

Elwood, J.M., et al. "Sunburn, suntan and the risk of cutaneous malignant melanoma: the Western Canada Melanoma study." *Br J Cancer* 1985; 35: 427.

Environment Canada. A Primer on Ozone Depletion. Ottawa, 1993.

Epstein, S.S. *The Politics of Cancer*. New York: Anchor Books, 1979.

————. "Evaluation of the national cancer program and proposed reforms." *Intl J Health Servs* 1993; 23: 15-44.

Flack, F., et al. "Pesticides and PCB residues in human breast lipids and their relation to breast cancer." *Archives Environ Hlth* 1992; 47: 143-146.

Farley, T.A., and J.T. Flannery. "Late-stage diagnosis of breast cancer in women of lower socioeconomic status: public health implications." *Am J Pub Hlth* 1989; 79: 1508-1512.

Frank, R., et al. "Organochlorine residues in adipose tissues, blood and milk from Ontario residents, 1976-1985." *Can J Pub Hlth* 79 (3): 150-158.

Funch, D.P. A Report on cancer survival in the economically disadvantaged. Prepared for the Am Cancer Society Subcommittee on Hlth Care of

Economically Disadvantaged Cancer Patients, 1985.

Funch, D.P. "Socioeconomic status and survival for breast and cervical cancer." *Women and Health* 1986; 11: 37-54.

Ghadirian, P., J.P. Thouez, and A. Simard. "La geographie du cancer de l'oesophage." *Soc Sci and Med* 1988; 27: 971-985.

Gottileb, M.S., et al., "Lung cancer in Louisiana: death certificate analysis." *J Natl Cancer Inst* 1979; 63, 1131-1137.

Gorham, B.D., C.F. Garland, and F.C. Garland. "Acid haze, air pollution and breast and cancer colon cancer mortality in twenty Canadian cities." *Can J Pub Hlth* 1989; 80: 96-100.

Griffith, J.L., et al. "Cancer mortality in U.S. counties with hazardous waste sites and environmental pollution." *Archives Environ Hlth* 1989; 44: 69-74.

Halpern, M.T., B.H.W. Gillespie, and K.E. Warner. "Patterns of absolute risk of lung cancer mortality in former smokers." *J Natl Cancer Inst* 1993; 85: 457-464.

Hancock, T. "Sustaining Health: Achieving Health for all in a Secure Environment." Paper presented at the Conference on Health-Environment-Economy, York Univ., Toronto, April 1989.

Hatch, M.C., et al. "Cancer rates after the Three Mile Island nuclear accident and proximity of residence to the plant." *Amer J Pub Hlth* 1991; 81: 719-724.

Hayes, H.M., et al. "Case control study of canine malignant lymphoma: positive association with dog owner's use 2,4-dichlorophenoxyacetic acid herbicides." *J Natl Cancer Inst* 1991; 83: 1226-1231.

Henriksen, T., et al. "Ultraviolet-radiation and skin cancer: effect of an ozone layer depletion." *Photochem Photobiol* 1990; 51: 579-582.

Horstman, D., W. McDonnell, et al. "Changes in pulmonary function and airway reactivity due to prolonged exposure to typical ambient ozone levels." In T. Schneider, et al., eds., *Atmospheric Ozone Research and its Policy Implications.* Amsterdam: Elsevier, 1989.

Howe, G.R., J.D. Burch, A.B. Miller, et al. "Tobacco use, occupation, coffee, various nutrients, and bladder cancer." *J Natl Cancer Inst* 1980; 64: 701-713.

Infante, P.F., and G.K. Puhl. "Living in a chemical world: actions and reactions to industrial carcinogens." *Teratogenesis Carcinog.* Mutagen 1988; 8: 225-249.

IARC. IARC Monographs on the Evaluation of Carcinogenic Risks of Chemicals to Humans. Vol 38, Tobacco smoke. Lyon: Intl Agency for Research on Cancer, 1986.

———. IARC Monographs on the Evaluation of Carcinogenic Risks of Chemicals to Humans. Suppl 7. Lyon: Intl Agency for Research on Cancer, 1987a.

———. IARC Monographs on the Evaluation of Carcinogenic Risks of Chemicals to Humans. Vol 42, Silica and some silicates. Lyon: Intl Agency for Research on Cancer, 1987b.

———. IARC Monographs on the Evaluation of Carcinogenic Risks of Chemicals to Humans. Vol 44. Alcohol drinking. Lyon: Intl Agency for Research on Cancer, 1988.

———. IARC Monographs on the Evaluation of Carcinogenic Risks of Chemicals to Humans. Vol 59. Hepatitis viruses. Lyon: Intl Agency for Research on Cancer, 1994.

———. IARC Monographs on the Evaluation of Carcinogenic Risks of Chemicals to Humans. Vol 60. Some industrial chemicals. Lyon: Intl Agency for Research on Cancer, 1994.

———. IARC Monographs on the Evaluation of Carcinogenic Risks of Chemicals to Humans. Vol 61. Schistosomes, liver flukes and Helicobacter pylori. Lyon: Intl Agency for Research on Cancer, 1994.

IARC Study Group on Cancer Risk among Nuclear Industry Workers. "Direct estimates of cancer mortality due to low doses of ionizing radiation: an international study." *Lancet* 1994; 34: 1039-1043.

Industrial Disease Standards Panel. Report to the Workers' Compensation Board on Lung Cancer in the Hardrock Mining Industry. IDSP Report No. 12, Toronto, 1994.

International Joint Commission. Sixth Biennial Report on Great Lakes Water Quality. Windsor, Ontario: International Joint Commission, 1992.

Jones, R.R. "Ozone depletion and cancer risk." *Lancet* 1987; 2: 443-446.

Kaldor, J.M., N.E. Day, and S. Shiboski. "Epidemiological studies of anticancer drug carcinogenicity." In Schmael, D., and J.M. Kaldor, eds., Carcinogenicity of alkylating cytostatic drugs. IARC scientific publications no 78. Lyon: Intl Agency for Research on Cancer, 1986; pp 189-201.

Keiding, L.M. "General preventive measures against carcinogenic exposure in the external environment." *Pharma and Toxic* 1993; 72 (Suppl 1), s136-s138.

Kendall, P. City of Toronto Dept Pub Hlth presentation to the Standing Committee on the Environment and Sustainable Development of the House of Commons. Toronto, Ontario 17, 1994.

Khlat, M. "Mortality from melanoma in migrants to Australia: variation by age of arrival and duration of stay." *Am. J Epidemiol* 1992; 135: 103.

Kjaer, S.K., P. Poll, H. Jensen, et al. "Abnormal Papanicolau smear. A population-based study of risk factors in Greenlandic and Danish women." *Acta Obstet Gynecol Scand* 1990; 69: 79-86.

Koutsky, L.A., D.A. Galloway, and K.K. Holmes. "Epidemiology of genital human papillomavirus infection." *Epidemio Reviews* 1988; 10: 122-163.

Kreiger, N., M.S. Wolff, R.A. Hiatt, et al. "Breast cancer and serum organochlorides: a prospective study among white, black and Asian women." *J Natl Cancer Inst* 1994; 86: 589-599.

Kusiak, R.A., J. Springer, et al. "Carcinoma of the lung in Ontario gold miners: possible aetiological factors." *Br J Ind Med* 1991; 48: 808-817.

Labonte, R., and K. Davies. "Stop the carcinogens." *Policy Options* 7, 33-57, 1986.

Landrigan, P.L. "Environmental disease: a preventable catastrophe." *Amer J Pub Hlth* 1992; 82: 941-943.

Leon, D.A. The Social Distribution of Cancer, Longitudinal Study 1971-1975. London: HMSO Series LS No. 3, 1988.

Letourneau, E.G., D. Krewski, N.W. Choi, et al. "Case-control study of residential radon and lung cancer in Winnipeg, Manitoba, Canada." *Am J Epidemiol* 1994; 140: 310-322.

Levi, F., et al. "Socioeconomic groups and cancer risk: a death at the Swiss Canton at Vaud." *Intl J Epidimiol* 1988; 17: 711-717.

Lindheim, R., and S.L. Syme. "Environments, people and health." *Ann Rev*

Pub Hlth 1983; 4: 335-359.

Longnecker, M.P. "Alcoholic beverage consumption in relation to risk of breast cancer: meta-analysis and review." *Cancer causes and control* 1994; 5: 73-82.

Maltoni, C., and I.J. Selikoff. "Living in a chemical world: occupational and environmental significance of industrial carcinogens." *Annals New York Acad Sci* 1988; 534: 1-1045.

Magano, J.J. "Cancer mortality near Oak Ridge, Tennessee." *Intl J Hlth Serv* 1994; 24: 521-533.

Marrett, L.D., et al. "The use of host factors to identify people at high risk for cutaneous malignant melanoma." *C Med Assoc J* 1992; 147: 445-453.

Martin, K.A., and M.W. Freeman. "Postmenopausal hormone-replacement therapy." *New Eng J Med* 1993; 328: 1115-1117.

McGinnis, J.M., and W.H. Foege. "Actual causes of death in the United States." *JAMA* 1993; 270: 2207-2212.

McWhorter, W.P., et al. "Contribution of socioeconomic status to black/white differences in cancer incidence." *Cancer* 1989; 63: 982-987.

Millar, J. "Sex differentials in mortality by income level in urban Canada." *Can J Pub Hlth* 1983; 74: 329-334.

Miller, A.B. "Asbestos fiber dust and gastro-intestinal malignancies. Review of literature with regard to a cause/effect relationship." *J Charon Dis* 1978; 31: 23-33.

———. "An overview of hormone-associated cancers." *Cancer Res* 1978; 38: 3985-3990.

———. "Risk/Benefit considerations of antiestrogen/estrogen therapy in healthy postmenopausal women." *Preventive Med* 1991; 20: 79-85.

———. "Planning cancer control strategies." *Chronic Diseases in Canada* 1992; 13 (1 Suppl), s1-s39.

Miller, A.B., G. Anderson, J. Brisson, et al. "Report of a National Workshop on Screening for Cancer of the Cervix." *Can Med Ass J* 1991; 145: 1301-1325.

Miller, A.B., F. Berrino, M. Hill, et al. "Diet in the aetiology of cancer: a review." *Eur J Cancer* 1994; 30A: 207-220.

Morris, R.D., et al. "Chlorination, chlorination by-products and cancer: a meta-analysis." *Amer J Publ Hlth* 1992; 82: 955-963.

Muir, C.S., and A.J. Sasco. "Prospects for cancer control in the 1990s." *Ann Rev Pub Hlth* 1990; 11: 143-163.

Mustard, J.F., E. Farber, A.B. Miller, D. McCalla, and J.E. Till. Report of the Special Advisory Committee on Carcinogens. Fourth Annual Report of the Advisory Council on Occup Hlth and Occup Safety, 1981-1982. 1982.

National Academy of Sciences. Potential Risk of Lung Cancer from Diesel Engine Emissions. Washington D.C.: National Academy Press, 1981.

National Academy of Sciences. Regulating Pesticides in Food: The Delaney Paradox. Washington D.C.: National Academy Press, 1987.

National Cancer Institute. Bioassay of Chlordane for Possible Carcinogenicity. Bethesda, Maryland: Carcinogenesis Technical Report Series 8, 1977.

National Cancer Institute of Canada. Canadian cancer statistics, 1995. Toronto, 1995.

National Coalition Against the Misuse of Pesticides (U.S.). Testimony of NCAMP before the Senate Subcommittee on Toxic Substances, Environmental Oversight, Research and Development, Committee on Environment and Public Works, 1981.

National Council of Welfare. Health, Health Care and Medicare: A Report by the National Council of Welfare. Ottawa: Ministry of Supply and Services, 1990.

National Institute for Occupational Safety and Health Carcinogenic Effects of Exposure to Diesel Exhaust. Bethesda, Maryland: NIOSH Current Intelligence Bulletin 50, 1988.

Nightingale, T.E., and J. Gruber. "Helicobacter and human cancer." *J Natl Cancer Inst* 1994; 86: 1505-1509.

Nsubuga, J. "Organochlorine residues and breast cancer risks in women." *PHERO* 1993; June 18, 170-172.

Onstot, J.R., R. Ayling, and J. Stanley. Characterization of HRRC/CCMS Unidentified Peaks from the Analysis of Human Adipose Tissue. Washington, D.C.: U.S. EPA 560 / 6-87-002a, 1987.

Ontario Fair Tax Commission Final Report of the Working Group on Environment and Taxation. Toronto: Queen's Printer for Ontario, 1992.

Ontario Hydro. Annual Summary and Assessment of Environmental Radiological Data for 1991. Toronto: Queen's Printer for Ontario, 1991.

Ontario Ministry of Agriculture and Food, and Ministry of the Environment. Polychlorinated dibenzo-p-dioxins and polychlorinated dibenzofurans and other organochlorine contaminants in food. Toronto: Queen's Printer for Ontario, 1988.

Ontario Ministry of Environment and Energy. Candidate Substances for Bans, Phase-Outs or Reductions. Toronto: Queen's Printer for Ontario, 1993.

Ontario Ministry of Health. A Guide for Community Health Promotion Planning. Toronto: Queen's Printer for Ontario, 1991.

Ozonoff, D. "Taking the Handle of the Chlorine Pump." Presentation made at Public Health Forum, Boston Univ School of Pub Hlth, October 5, 1993.

Pearce, N.E., and J.K. Howard. "Occupation, social class and male cancer mortality in New Zealand 1974-78." *Int J Epid* 1986; 15: 456-462.

Premier's Council on Health, Well-Being and Social Justice. Our Environment Our Health: Report of the Review Committee on Goal 3. Toronto: Queen's Printer for Ontario, 1993.

Preston, D.S., and R.S. Stern. "Nonmelanoma Cancers of the skin." *N Eng J. Med* 1992; 327: 1649-1661.

Pukkala, E., and L. Teppo. "Socioeconomic Status and Education as risk determinants of gastrointestinal cancer." *Prev Med* 1986; 15: 127-138.

Qureshi, A.M., and H.E. Robertson. "Polychlorinated byphenyls (PCB) in breast milk from Regina nursing mothers." *Can J Pub Hlth* 1987; 78: 389-392.

Rabkin, C.S., and F. Yellin. "Cancer incidence in a population with a high prevalence of infection with human immunodeficiency virus type 1." *J Natl Cancer Inst* 1994; 86: 1711-1716.

Rall, D. "Laboratory animal toxicity and carcinogensis testing: underlying concepts, advances and constraints." *Annals New York Acad Sci* 1988; 534: 78-83.

Raloff, J. "That feminine touch." Science News 1994; 145, 56-59.

Rimpela, A.H., and E.I. Pukkala. "Cancers of affluence: positive social class gradient and rising incidence trend in some cancer forms." Soc Sci Med 1987; 24: 601-606.

Risch H.A, L.D. Marrett, and G.R. Howe. "Parity, contraception, infertility, and the risk of ovarian cancer." Amer J Epidemio 1994; 140: 585-597.

Romieu, I., J.A. Berlin, and G. Colditz. "Oral contraceptives and breast cancer. Review and meta-analysis." Cancer 1990; 66:2253-2263.

Rundall, T., and W. Bruvold. "A meta-analysis of school-based smoking and alcohol use prevention programs." Hlth Educ Quarterly 1988; 15:317-334.

Samet, J.M. "Indoor radon and lung cancer: risk or not? J Natl Cancer Inst 1994; 86:1813-1814.

Schiffman, M.H., H.M. Bauer, R.N. Hoover, et al. "Epidemiologic evidence showing that human pappillomavirus infection causes most cervical intraepithelial neoplasia." J Natl Cancer Inst 1993; 85:958-964.

Scribner, J.D., and N.K. Mottett. "DDT acceleration of mammary gland tumors induced in the male Sprague-Dewey rate by 2-acetamio-phenanthrene." Carcinogensis 2; 1236-1239, 1981.

Shames, L.S., M.T. Munekata, and M.C. Pike. "Re: Blood levels of organochlorine residues and risk of breast cancer." J Natl Cancer Inst 1994; 86:1642-1643.

Shannon, H.S., et al. "Lung cancer and air pollution in an industrial city— a geographical analysis." Can J Pub Hlth 1988; 79: 255-259.

Shimikawa, T., P. Soblie, M.A. Carpenter, et al. "Dietary intake patterns and sociodemographic factors in the atherosclerosis risk in communities study." Prev Med 1994; 12:769-780.

Small, B., et al. Healthy Environments of Canadians. Ottawa: Health and Welfare Canada.

Stern, R.S., et al. "Risk reduction for nonmelanoma skin cancer with childhood sunscreen use." Arch Dermatol 1986; 122: 537-545.

Swerdlow, A.J., J. English, and R.M. Mackie. "Benign nevi associated with high risk of cutaneous malignant melanoma." Lancet 1984; 11:168-170.

Surgeon General. The health consequences of involuntary smoking.

Washington, D.C.: U.S. Dept of Health and Human Services, 1986.

The Alpha-Tocopherol, Beta Caroten Cancer Prevention Study Group. "The effect of vitamin B and beta carotene on the incidence of lung cancer and other cancers in smokers." *N Engl J Med* 1994; 330: 1029-1035.

Theriault, G., M. Goldberg, A.B. Miller, et al. "Cancer risks associated with occupational exposure to magnetic fields among electric utility workers in Ontario and Quebec, Canada and France: 1970-1989." *Am J Epidemiol* 1994; 139:550-572.

Thomas, D.B. "Oral contraceptives and breast cancer." *J Natl Cancer Inst* 1993; 85:359-364.

Thompson, S.C., D. Jolley, and R. Marks. "Reduction of solar keratoses by regular sunscreen use." *New Eng J Med* 1993; 329: 1147-1151.

Thornton, J. Chlorine, Human Health and the Environment; The Breast Cancer Warning. Washington, D.C.: Greenpeace, 1993.

Tomatis, L., A. Aitio, N.E. Day, E. Heseltine, et al. Cancer: Causes, Occurrence and Control. Lyon: IARC Scientific Publications No. 100, 1990.

Upton, A.C., T. Kneip, and P. Toniolo. "Public health aspects of toxic chemical disposal sites." *Ann Rev Pub Hlth* 1989; 10: 1-25.

U.S. Dept of Health and Human Services and U.S. Environmental Protection Agency. Respiratory health effects of passive smoking: Lung cancer and other disorders. The Report of the U.S. Environmental Protection Agency. Smoking and Control Monograph 4. NIH Publication No. 93-3605, 1993.

U.S. Public Health Service. "Even some exercise offers health benefits." Prevention Report October/November 1994, 1,2,4.

Vineis, P., and L. Simonato. "Estimates of the proportion of bladder cancers attributable to occupation." *Scand J Work Environ Hlth*, 1986; 12:55-60.

Vitasa, B.C., et al. "Association of non-melanoma skin cancer and actinic keratosis and cumulative solar ultraviolet exposure in Maryland waterman." *Cancer* 1990; 65: 2811-2817.

Walker, A.I.T., et al. "The toxicology and pharmacodynamics of dieldrin: two year oral exposure of rats and dogs." *Toxicology and Applied Pharmac* 1969; 15: 345-373.

Wasserman, M., et al. "Organochlorine compounds in neoplastic and adjacent apparently normal breast tissue." *Bulletin Environ Contaminants and Toxicology* 1976; 15: 478-484.

Webster, T. "Dioxin and human health: a public health assessment of dioxin exposure in Canada." Unpublished manuscript. Boston: Boston Univ School of Pub Hlth, 1994.

Westin, J.B., and E. Richter. "The Israeli breast cancer anomaly." *Ann. New York Acad Sci* 1990; 609: 269-279.

Whitehead, M. The Health Divide. London: Health Education Council, 1987.

Wigle, D.T., R.M. Semenciw, K. Wilkins, et al. "Mortality study of Canadian male farm operators: non-Hodgkins lymphoma and agricultural practices in Saskatchewan." *J Natl Cancer Inst* 1990; 82: 575-582.

Willett, W. Presentation to the President's Cancer Panel. April, 1994.

Wilson, P.D., K.H. Kaldbey, and A.M. Kligman. "Ultraviolet light sensitivity and prolonged UVR-erythema." *J Invest Dermatol* 1981; 77: 434-436.

Windsor Air Quality Committee. "Windsor air quality study." Toronto; Science and Technology Branch, Ministry of Environment and Energy, 1994.

Wolff, M.S., P.G. Toniolo, E.W. Lee, et al. "Blood levels of organochlorine residues and risk of breast cancer." *J Natl Cancer Inst* 1993; 85: 648-652.

The WHO Collaborative Study of Neoplasia and Steroid Contraceptives. "Depo-medroxyprogesterone acetate (DMPA) and risk of endometrial cancer." *Intl J Cancer* 1991; 49: 186-190.

World Health Organization. Ottawa Charter for Health Promotion. Ottawa, 1986.

Secondary Sources

"10 Tips To Healthy Eating." American Dietetic Association and National Center for Nutrition and Dietetics (NCND), April 1994.

1997 Research Report, from CCFA National Scientific Advisory Committee, Division of Digestive Diseases, Univ of North Carolina, Chapel Hill, posted to: MedicineNet, Information Network, Inc. 1997.

Action on Smoking and Health. Pipe and cigar smoking: The report of an expert group appointed by Action on Smoking and Health. *Practitioner* 1973;210:645–648.

Antibiotics in Animals: An Interview with Stephen Sundlof, D.V.M., Ph.D." International Food Information Council, 1100 Connecticut Avenue N.W., Suite 430, Washington, D.C. 20036, 1997.

Arsenault, Gillian, M.D., Breast Cancer Epidemiology, unpublished report, 1996.

Ayanian, John Z., Betsy A. Kohler, Toshi Abe, and Arnold M. Epstein. "The relation between health insurance coverage and clinical outcomes among women with breast cancer." *New Engl J Med*, Vol 329, No 5 (29 July 1993): 326-331.

Bailar, John C. III, and Heather Gornick. "Cancer Undefeated." *New Engl J Med*, May 29, 1997, 336(22):1569-74.

Bartlett, J.G. Epidemiology and clinical aspects of antibiotic-associated colitis. Proceedings of the 2nd International Symposium on Anaerobes, June 22, 1985, Tokyo.

Batt, Sharon. *Patient No More: The Politics of Breast Cancer*. Charlottetown, PEI: gynergy books, 1994.

Benowitz, N.L. "Pharmacologic aspects of cigarette smoking and nicotine addiction." *New Engl J Med* 1988; 319:1318-1330.

Berndl, Leslie, R.D. "Understanding Fat." *Diabetes Dialogue* (Vol 42, No 1) Spring 1995.

Bernstein, Leslie, and Jennifer L. Kelsey. "Epidemiology and Prevention of Breast Cancer." Dept of Health Research and Policy, Stanford Univ, and Dept of Preventive Med, Univ of Southern Calif (1996): 47-67.

Bertell, Rosalie. Links between ionizing radiation and breast cancer. Paper presented at the World Conference on Breast Cancer, July13-17, 1997, Kingston, Ontario.

Beyers, Joanne. "How sweet it is!" *Diabetes Dialogue* (Vol 42, No 1) Spring 1995.

Bondy, M., and C. Mastromarino. "Ethical issues of genetic testing and their implications in epidemiologic studies." *Annals of Epidemio*, July, 1997, Vol 7: 363-366.

Bove, C.M., et al. "Presymptomatic and predisposition genetic testing:ethical and social considerations." *Semin Oncol Nurs* 1997 May 13:135-140.

Britt, Beverley, Dr. "Pesticides and Alternatives." Excerpted from the Canadian Organic Growers Toronto Chapter's Spring Conference:1-4.

Brody, J., et al. Mapping the history of pesticide use in the Cape Cod Breast Cancer and Environment Study. Paper presented at the World Conference on Breast Cancer, July13-17, 1997, Kingston, Ontario.

Busby, Chris, Dr. The current increase in breast cancer trend worldwide has its origin in ionizing radiation exposure to components of global weapons testing fallout. Paper presented at the World Conference on Breast Cancer, July13-17, 1997, Kingston, Ontario.

"Calories Count In Colon Cancer Risk" *Amer J Epidemio*, 1997;145:199-210.

"A Cancer Gene Makes Colon Removal An Option." *The New York Times*, March 19, 1997.

"Cancer In Massachusetts Town Cause By Demographics, Not Environment" *Boston Globe*, Jan 15, 1997 02:01 AM EST.

Caplan, L.S. "Disparities in breast cancer screening: is it ethical?" *Pub Hlth Rev* 1997, Vol 25: 31-41.

Casstevens, Rebecca. Addressing current uses of pesticides linked with breast cancer. Paper presented at the World Conference on Breast Cancer, July13-17, 1997, Kingston, Ontario.

Centre For Health Promotion, Dept of Public Health Sciences, Univ of Toronto. Proceedings of a Conference on The Effect of Hormonal Disrupters on the Health and Development of Children, June 25, 1999.

Chaddock, Brenda, CDE, "Activity is key to diabetes health." *Can Pharm J*, March 1997.

———. "Foul Weather Fitness: The hardest part is getting started." *Can Pharm J*, March 1996.

———. "The Magic of Exercise." *Can Pharm J*, September 1995.

———. "The Right Way to Read a Label." *Can Pharm J*, May 1996.

"Chemical in Green Tea Stops Tumors, Study Says." Reuters, Thursday, June

5 2:01 AM EDT.

Colborn, Theo, J.P. Myers, and Dianne Dumanoski, *Our Stolen Future*. New York: Dutton, 1996.

Colorectal Cancer Screening. Final Report of the Ontario Expert Panel, April 1999.

Dickens, Bernard M., Nancy Pei, and Kathryn M. Taylor. "Legal and Ethical Issues in Genetic Testing and Counseling for Susceptibility to Breast, Ovarian and Colon Cancer." *Can Med Assn J*, March 15, 1996; 154 (6):813-818.

Doan, Brian D., et al. Psychological issues facing high risk women seeking genetic testing for hereditary breast cancer. Paper presented at the World Conference on Breast Cancer, July 13-17, 1997, Kingston, Ontario.

"Editorial, Exercise and Breast Cancer—Time to Get Moving?" *New Engl J Med*, May 1, 1997, Vol 336, No 18.

Eighth Biennial Report On Great Lakes Water Quality, Under the Great Lakes Water Quality Agreement of 1978 to the Governments of the United States and Canada and the State and Provincial Governments of the Great Lakes Basin. Intl Joint Commission, 1250 23rd Street NW, Suite 100, Washington, D.C. 20440. 1996.

Engel, June V. "Beyond Vitamins: Phytochemicals to help fight disease." *Health News*, June 1996, Vol 14, Univ of Toronto.

————. "Eating Fiber." *Diabetes Dialogue*, (Vol 44, No 1) Spring 1997.

"Engineering a treatment for Crohn's disease." *Lancet*, Vol 349, No 9051, Saturday 22 February 1997.

Environmental and Occupational Working Groups of the Toronto Cancer Prevention Coalition. Preventing Cancer From Environmental and Occupational Factors: A Strategy for the City of Toronto. Executive Summary, March 7, 2000, by CAW Canada, Cancer In Your Workplace: A Manual For Worker Investigators.

Environmental Health Program of the Environmental Defense Fund. Executive Report, 1997.

Epstein, Samuel S.,and David Steinmean with Suzanne LeVert, *The Breast Cancer Prevention Program: The First Complete Survey of the Causes of Breast Cancer and the Steps You Can Take to Reduce Your Risks*. New York:

Macmillan, 1998.

Esserman, Dr. Laura. "Breast cancer gene screening for at-risk women." posted online @ www.mediconsult.com/breast/news, November 8, 1998.

"Estrogen Gene Tied To Breast Cancer Risk," *The New York Times*, March 26, 1997.

Everyday Carcinogens: Stopping Cancer Before It Starts. Proceedings from the March 1999 Workshop on Primary Cancer Prevention, McMaster Univ, Hamilton, Ontario.

"Evidence for Estrogen." *Med Post*, 9 April 1996:75-76.

Farquhar, Andrew. "Exercising essentials." *Diabetes Dialogue* (Vol 43, No 3) Fall 1996: 6-8.

"Fat, Alcohol Increase Breast Cancer Risk," Reuters. *Epidemiology* (1997;8:425-428), Monday June 16 6:14 PM EDT.

Feldman, Gayle. "Is Genetic Testing Right For You?" *Self*. October 1996:187-209.

Fletcher, S.W. "Whither scientific deliberation in health policy recommendations? Alice in the wonderland of breast-cancer screening." *N Engl J Med* 1997;336:1180-83.

————. "Confusion about Breast-Cancer Screening." *N Engl J Med* 1997; 336:1465-71.

Food and Drug Administration. "Nutrient Claims Guide for Individual Foods." Special Report, Focus On Food Labeling. FDA Publication No. 95-2289.

"Food and Exercise: Guidelines to a Healthier You." Patient information. Bayer Inc. Healthcare Division, 1997.

Fox, Maggie, "Researchers Show How Genes Fail In Breast Cancer." Reuters, April 23, 1997 7:02 p.m. EDT.

Fraser, Eliabeth, and Bill Clarke. "Loafing Around." *Diabetes Dialogue* (Vol 44, No 1) Spring 1997.

From Policy To Action. Symposium by the Toronto Cancer Prevention Coalition, March 7-8, 2000.

"Getting to the Roots of a Vegetarian Diet," Vegetarian Resource Group,

Baltimore, Maryland, 1997.

Gilbert, Susan. "Doctors often misread results of genetic tests, study finds," *The New York Times*, March 26, 1997.

Gofman, John W. Preventing Breast Cancer: The Story of a Major, Proven, Preventable Cause of This Disease. (1995, CNR Book Division, Committee for Nuclear Responsibility, San Francisco, CA.)

Habib, Marlene. "Low-fat diet and exercise reduce breast cancer risk," *Canadian Press*, January 10, 1997.

Habib, Marlene. "Pollution seen as chief culprit in breast cancer: 80 per cent of cases tied to ecology mishaps." *Winnipeg Free Press*, July 17, 1997.

Harrison, Pam. "Rethinking obesity." *Family Practice*, March 11, 1996.

Health Symposium Addresses Breast Cancer and Obesity. Scripps-McClatchy, Western. Feb 2, 1997 01:01 AM EST.

Healy, Bernadette. "BRCA Genes—Bookmaking, Fortunetelling, and Medical Care." *New Engl J Med*, 336(20): 1448-1449: May 15, 1997.

Hendler, Saul Sheldon. *The Doctors' Vitamin and Mineral Encyclopedia*. New York: Fireside Books, 1990.

"Hereditary breast cancer in the Jewish population." Mount Sinai Hospital, November 1996.

Hill, D., V. White, and N. Gray. "Australian patterns of tobacco smoking in 1989." *Med J Aust* 1991; 154:797–801.

Hilts, Philip. "Risks of Colon Cancer," *The New York Times*, April 24, 1997.

Hislop, Gregory T. "The Role of Nutrition in the Prevention of Cancer." *Can J CME*, March 1995:111-118.

Ho, Marian. "Learning Your ABCs, Part Two." *Diabetes Dialogue* (Vol 43, No 3) Fall 1996.

Holowaty, Phillippa. "Breast Cancer Gene Research." Presented to The Alliance of Breast Cancer Survivors, November 13, 1997.

Holtzman, N.A. "Medical and ethical issues in genetic screening—an academic view." *Environ Health Perspect* 1996 Oct 104 Suppl 5: 987-990.

Hoy, Claire. *The Truth About Breast Cancer*. Toronto: Stoddart, 1995.

Hunter, J.E., and T.H. Applewhite. "Reassessment of Trans Fatty Acid Availability in the U.S. Diet." *Am J Clin Nutr* 54:363-9, 1991.

Hurley, Jane, and Stephen Schmidt. "Going with the Grain." *Nutrition Action*, October 1994:10-11.

Immen, Wallace. "Repeated dieting may raise cancer risk. Chemicals stored in fat spur rapid growth and may increase chances of mutations in cells," *The Globe and Mail*, April 16, 1997.

International Agency of Research on Cancer. IARC Monograph on the Evaluation of Carcinogenic Risk of Chemicals to Humans. Tobacco Smoking. Switzerland: World Health Organisation, 1986:38.

Ionescu, Simona-Adriana. Causes of breast and colon cancer in Romania. Paper presented at the World Conference on Breast Cancer, July13-17, 1997, Kingston, Ontario.

Kea, David. "Herd Health: The biggest reward of ecological dairy farming." *Cognition*, Winter 1992/93:26-27.

Kishi, Misa. Impact of pesticides on health in developing countries: Research, policy and actions. Paper presented at the World Conference on Breast Cancer, July13-17, 1997, Kingston, Ontario.

Kock, Henry. "Restoring Natural Vegetation as Part of the Farm." Gardening without Chemicals '91, Canadian Organic Growers Toronto Chapter, 6 April 1991.

Kolata, Gina. "Ticking Bomb: The Presence of a Breast-Cancer Gene Creates Other Problems For Some Women.," *The New York Times*, Sunday, March 2, 1997.

Kuczmarski, R.J., K.M. Flegal, S.M. Campbell, and C.L. Johnson. "Increasing Prevalence of Overweight Among U.S. Adults: The National Health and Nutrition Examination Surveys, 1960 to 1991. *J Amer Med Assn*, 272:205-211, 1994.

Levine, R.J. *Ethics and Regulation of Clinical Research*. New Haven: Yale University Press, 1988.

Liebman, Bonnie. "Walking and Cancer." *Nutrition Action*, March 1998:13.

Mangano, Joseph J. Breast cancer from radioactive emissions by nuclear power plants in Connecticut, USA. Paper presented at the World Conference on Breast Cancer, July13-17, 1997, Kingston, Ontario.

Mastroianni, Anna C., Ruth Faden, and Daniel Federman, eds., *Women and Health Research: Ethical and Legal Issues of Including Women in Clinical Studies*, Vol 1. Washington: National Academy Press, 1994.

McAuliffe, Kathleen. "Dying of Embarrassment." *More*, May/June, 1999:52-62.

Meen, Elizabeth, "Ex-Bell employees uncover high levels of cancer at Hamilton office." *The Expositor*, May 7, 1998.

Minister of Health, Minister of Public Works and Government Services Canada. State of Knowledge Report on Environmental Contaminants and Human Health in the Great Lakes Basin. Catalogue Number H46-2/97-214E, 1997.

O'Connell, Peter, Vladimir Pekkel, Suzanne A. W. Fuqua, et al. "Molecular genetic studies of early breast cancer evolution by LOH," retrieved online from www.mars.uthscsa.edu/Publications/MGSEBCE/ mgsebce.html, February 16, 1999.

"Oats are in." Countdown USA: Countdown to a Healthy Heart, Allegheny General Hospital and Voluntary Hospitals of America, Inc., 1990.

"Olestra: yes or no?" Excerpted from *Univ of Calif at Berkley Wellness Letter*, c. Health Associates, *Diabetes Dialogue* (Vol 43, No 3) Fall 1996.

Parens, Erik. "Glad and Terrified: On the Ethics of BRCA1 and 2 Testing." *Cancer Investigation*, 14(4), 405-411, 1996.

Patient Information. The National Digestive Diseases Information Clearinghouse (NDDIC), a service of the National Institute of Diabetes and Digestive and Kidney Diseases, part of the National Institutes of Health, under the U.S. Public Health Service. 1996, Licensed to Medical Strategies, Inc.

"Putting fun back into food," International Food Information Council, 1100 Connecticut Avenue N.W., Suite 430, Washington, D.C. 20036, 1997.

"Q&A about Fatty Acids and Dietary Fats." International Food Information Council 1100 Connecticut Avenue N.W., Suite 430, Washington, D.C. 20036, 1997.

Quigley, Ann. "Group recommends banning baking additive." Reuters Health, July 21, 1999.

Rebbeck, T.R., F.J. Couch, J. Kant, et al. "Genetic heterogeneity in hereditary breast cancer: role of BRCA1 and BRCA2." *Am J Hum Genet*. 1996 59(3): 547-553.

Reilly, P.R., et al. "Ethical issues in genetic research: disclosure and informed consent." *Nat Genet* 1997 Jan 15: 16-20.

"Relation of Breast Cancer with Passive and Active Exposure to Tobacco Smoke." *Amer J Epidemio* (Vol 143, No 9): 918, 927.

Rifkin, Jeremy. "Playing God with the Genetic Code." *Health Naturally*, April/May 1995: 40-44

Robson, Barbara. "Conferences Point to Growing Concern about Possible Links Between Breast Cancer, Environment." *Can Med Assn J* 8 (154; 15 April 1996): 1254.

Rosenthal, M. Sara. *Managing Your Diabetes*. Toronto: Macmillan Canada, 1998.

———. *The Breast Sourcebook*, 2nd ed. Los Angeles: Lowell House, 1999.

———. *The Gastrointestinal Sourcebook*. Los Angeles: Lowell House,1997, 1999.

———. *The Gynecological Sourcebook*, 3rd ed. Chicago: Lowell House/ NTC, 1999.

Rudd, Dr. Wm. Warren, *Advice From The Rudd Clinic: A Guide To Colorectal Health*. Toronto: Macmillan Canada, 1997.

Safe, Stephen H. "Xenoestrogens and Breast Cancer." *New Engl J of Med* October 30, 1997, Vol 337, No 18.

Schreiber, Tatiana. "Misleading and Irresponsible: Cancer Activists Decry Harvard Report." *Resist*, April 1997.

"Scientific study explores role of dietary fat in breast cancer." Retrieved online from www.media.wayne.edu/iws.back.issues/iws3_20_97/breast_cancer.html, January 5, 1999.

"Scientists find new breast cancer gene." Reuters, March 1, 1998.

Seto, Carol. "Nutrition Labeling—U.S. style." *Diabetes Dialogue* (Vol 42, No 1) Spring 1995.

Sherwin, Susan. *Patient No Longer: Feminist Ethics and Health Care*.

Philadelphia: Temple University Press, 1984.

Shimer, Porter. *Keeping Fitness Simple: 500 Tips for fitting exercise into your life*. (1998, Storey Books, Pownal Vermont).

Simone, Rose, "Cancer link to workplace probed." *Kitchener-Waterloo Record*, May 10, 1998.

"Sorting Out the Facts About Fat," International Food Information Council 1100 Connecticut Avenue N.W., Suite 430, Washington, D.C. 20036, 1997.

Soto, Ana M., et al. "p-Nonyl-Phenol: An estrogenic xenobiotic released from 'modified' polystyrene." *Environ Hlth Perspectives*, Vol 92 (1991): 167-173.

Spake, Amanda. "Our Worst Fears About Pesticides and Plastics May Be Coming True—If Maverick Researcher Devra Lee Davis Is Right." 1995 *HEALTH* magazine, Document ID: MASO95C.

Sponselli, Christina, "Genetic testing raises questions." *Nurseweek*, November 1997.

————. "RNs can answer questions about genetics." *Nurseweek*, November 1997.

Stehlin, Dori. "A Little Lite Reading" posted to FDA website: www.fda.gov/fdac/foodlabel/diabetes.html. Retrieved online January 11, 1999.

Steingraber, Sandra. *Living Downstream: An Ecologist Looks At Cancer and the Environment*. New York: Addison-Wesley, 1997.

Stone, D.H., and S. Stewart. "Screening and the new genetics; a public health perspective on the ethical debate." *J Pub Hlth Med* 1996 Mar Vol 18:3-5.

Struewing, Jeffery P., et al. "The Risk of Cancer Associated with Specific Mutations of BRCA1 and BRCA2 among Ashkenazi Jews." *New Engl J Med*, May 15, 1997;336 (20):1401-1408.

Thune, Inger, et al. "Physical Activity and the Risk of Breast Cancer." *New Engl J Med*, May 1, 1997, Vol 336, No 18:1269-75.

"To Test Or Not To Test: The Debate Over Cancer-Gene Testing." *Salt Lake Tribune*, Feb 11, 1997 00:30 AM EST.

"Update on the Ontario Task Force on the Primary Prevention of Cancer," City of Toronto Public Health Dept, May 16, 1996.

U.S. Department of Health and Human Services. Reducing the Health Consequences of Smoking: 25 Years of Progress. A report of the Surgeon General. Rockville, Maryland: U.S. Department of Health and Human Services, Centre for Disease Control, Centre for Chronic Disease Prevention and Health Promotion, Office on Smoking and Health, 1989.

U.S. Department of Health and Human Services. The Health Consequences of Smoking: Cancer. A report of the Surgeon General. Rockville, Maryland: U.S. Department of Health and Human Services, Public Health Service, Office on Smoking and Health, 1982.

U.S. Department of Health and Human Services. The Health Consequences of Smoking: Chronic Obstructive Lung Disease. A report of the Surgeon General. Rockville, Maryland: U.S. Department of Health and Human Services, Public Health Service, Office on Smoking and Health, 1984.

U.S. Department of Health and Human Services. The Health Consequences of Smoking: Cardiovascular Disease. A report of the Surgeon General. Rockville, Maryland: U.S. Department of Health and Human Services, Public Health Service, Office on Smoking and Health, 1983.

Weijer, Charles. "Our Bodies, Our Science." The Sciences, May/June, 1995:41-45.

"What You Should Know About Sugars." International Food Information Council, 1100 Connecticut Avenue N.W., Suite 430, Washington D.C. 20036, May 1994.

Willett, W.C., et al. "Intake of Trans Fatty Acids and Risk of Coronary Heart Disease Among Women." Lancet 341:581-5, 1993.

"Wok cooking linked to lung cancer risk." Reuters Health, Aug 19, 1999

Wormworth, Janice. "Toxins and Tradition: The Impact of Food-Chain Contamination on the Inuit of Northern Quebec." Can Med Assn J (Vol 152, No 8), 15 April 1995.

ISBN 155212746-X